Health 4 You: An Easy to Use, Comprehensive Guide to Cooking, Eating and Surviving in Today's World

By Kevin Van Kirk

With Martin F. Perez

purposes, should be read or viewed for entertainment purposes only, and as a work of fiction.

Adherence to all applicable laws and regulations, both federal, state and local, governing professional licensing, business practices, advertising and all other aspects of doing business in the United States, or any other jurisdiction is the sole responsibility of the purchaser or reader.

Publisher: ToDoBlue Press

ISBN: 978-0-615-52832-8

Author: Kevin Van Kirk

Website: www.GodsFoodNow.com

Table of Contents:

Introduction

America has become a nation of sports-drink, Cheetos eating, fast food drive-in, buffet eating, "super-size me" addicted people. And we kind of love it – until we get on the scale and realize what we are doing to ourselves. That is, if you even have a scale in your home. At its most basic denominator, in today's culture there is a growing inability for restraint, good decision-making and correct perspectives when it comes to eating right. All you have to do to see this lack of restraint clearly, is to look around at how people live and eat today. The evidences of our lack of self-control can be shown in how unhealthy we are, what kills us (mortality rates), and how much our diet has changed for the worse over the last few years in particular. In America alone the Centers for Disease Control and Prevention published that in 2007 and 2008, 34% percent of adults ages 20 and older were considered obese. Obese is defined typically, as a person who is 20% over their ideal weight. More specifically, a person who has a Body Mass Index (BMI) of 30 and above is considered obese. Several factors are taken into account including height, age, sex and build. Along with those 34%, another 34% of adults over the age of 20 were also considered *over weight but not obese.* That amounts to over 66% (2/3rds of the adult population) over the age of 20 who have some weight struggle. As a comparison, in 1988 only 19% of adults over the age of 20 were considered obese. And that is simply looking at who we are via a weight perspective. There are others to measure including health and quality of life. You see, often people focus on weight as the primary indicator of a healthy person...but the fact of the matter is, you can be thin and equally or more unhealthy.

Looking further at our dieting make-up we see a grave trend in health, or shall I say more appropriately, our death. By far, heart disease and cancer lead mortality causes. The next closest cause of natural (or unnatural, if you prefer) death is stroke, at only 1/5 that of cancer deaths – cancer is second most. Heart disease's main cause is from...you guessed it...eating incorrectly. Heart disease is typically caused by Atherosclerosis, or a narrowing of the heart passages. And that is due primarily to the build-up of fatty cholesterol on the arterial wall. Cholesterol can only be found in animal product. The main reason people get heart disease: lack of exercise, bad diet, alcohol consumption, smoking and obesity.

We, as a nation, tend to walk around with the "well, it's the best I can do" mentality to health. We eat whatever is promoted enough on television, and then wonder why we aren't feeling all that hot. We eat low nutrition, high calorie foods and then wonder why we aren't losing any weight. Or why we can't fit into those jeans we used to wear in college. (As a side note, we probably shouldn't have ever worn jeans that small to begin with!) It's as though we have decided as a nation of people that it's okay to be a "chubby hubby", or gain the freshmen fifteen, or to get some love handles….after all, everyone is doing it. But is that really what we, what you, desire out of life? Or do you really, secretly, desire to get to or back to a better, more comfortable life?

It's no surprise then that we are growing more and more desperate for real answers to managing our eating habits…we're in effect, dying to know the right answers. Of course, if the main reason we are dying is due to poor diet and eating habits you'd expect that we'd be fighting every day to eat better and exercise more! But the reality is that we aren't. Instead, as a culture we just wait around for something to happen. For someone to tell us the truth and then make it happen for us. It's a real paradox. We scramble for answers but close our eyes in the process. Well…I'm here to help you do one thing: to help you open your eyes to what good health can be and perhaps help you gain a few years of quality life with insights into health and fitness! Every single person can get healthier. It's up to you where you will be. Continue reading as I not only share how to begin to make changes that can impact your life in a real way. But watch as I share with you a comprehensive approach to better eating, healthier lifestyles and durable, reliable and proven methods to gaining your life back.

This recipe book will provide an instruction manual to better eating and greater health, including recipes, meal planners, what to buy and even how much to buy! You'll get the insider tips to making the right types of meals and the support you desire in getting the weight off naturally and keeping it off realistically.

Of course, the first "secret" I'm going to share with you isn't a secret at all. There is no magic pill, no cure-all that takes no effort, no "easy as pie" shake or insta-anything that will make you healthier as you sit back and relax. Instead, you're going to get real advice from a man who knows the truth. You'll get the facts, the tools and the knowledge to do things right for long term health. I'm going to tell you that there are ways to lose weight immediately, within a day or two. But I don't want you to use those techniques. I want you to grow with me so that you can see the benefits of a change in lifestyle that will suit you well, and have you gain the energy, health and ability to live better.

***

The fact is, for 48 years I lived the standard American diet (SAD). I grew up on a ranch in southern Arizona where we raised beef, chickens and pigs to eat. My mother was a state fair champion in homemade breads. We worked hard and ate great, or so I thought. Once I got married, my wife made most all our meals from scratch. She always had vegetables or a salad on the plate. I ate a healthy SAD diet. At about 30 years old I began having bad chest pains. I went to the hospital thinking that I was having "the big one." They told me that I had a hiatus hernia and acid reflux. They put me on several different medications to coat my throat and reduce acids in my stomach. At the time I didn't realize that this was causing my systems to create even more acid to make up for the medications that were lowering the PH in my stomach. After all, that was what the doctors told me to do. I trusted the doctors.

Not so incidentally, I was also drinking about 5 diet sodas a day. It was supposed to help me lose some of the weight that I had started adding to my physique. At the time I didn't realize that the sodas were so acidic that they were leaching my bones of calcium trying to correct the acid PH from the sodas. Again -that was what the doctors told me to do. I trusted the doctors.

One fateful day, I was in a bad car accident on the freeway and tore some ligaments in my lower back. I went to the doctor and he prescribed some pain medication and anti-inflammatory pills. The doctors told me that the ligaments could not heal and as a result, I should take the meds. At the time I didn't realize that the medication was poisoning my body with huge amounts of toxins.

After being on the acid reflux meds, the pain meds and the diet sodas for awhile I started getting sick a lot...A LOT. My bones began hurting all the time. I would take more pain meds to deal with the pain. I went back to the doctor and he prescribed some heavy duty antibiotics to help me. At the time I did not realize that, not to put too fine a point on it, this was killing my immune system and setting me up for more serious problems down the road. I trusted the doctors.

You see, I was starting to get confused about this time of my life. My wife never went to the doctor, never took even aspirin and she was seldom sick. I was always on some new antibiotic, pain med, NSAD, or whatever the doctors would prescribe me. And I wasn't getting any better. I kind of felt like one of those little puppies that look out the storefront window at the people passing by – likely wondering why they don't have as good a life as the people walking by. I kept wondering why it was my wife who had better health than I did. I remember one day I was in severe pain from my bones hurting. My wife suggested that I stop drinking all the diet soda and maybe, just maybe that would help. She had read somewhere that the soda is extremely acidic and that can cause bone pain. After about 2 months and a few colon cleanses, the bone pain actually went away. I chalked it up to good luck on her part. I mean, she wasn't a doctor. What could she know, right?

Life went on this way for the next 15 years or so, with me eating the SAD diet, grabbing fast food more and more. I was busy and had things to do. I always compromised my eating in favor of time. Sound familiar? At any rate, I found myself 40 years old and almost 40 pounds overweight. I had been watching my blood pressure go up every year along with my weight. Strangely enough the doctors were now not as nice as they used to be. They said that I needed to get more serious. I needed to be on cholesterol meds and blood pressure meds. My wife, on her part was now trying harder and harder to get me to eat this Hallelujah diet way that she had read about some years back. I personally had begun studying vitamins to see if this might be the golden answer - that ever elusive "magic pill" that I needed. The more I studied the more I believed that I had found the crutch that I needed to continue my SAD eating habits. I figured this all-in-one vitamin stuff would be so much better than those meds. The result was that I started taking about $200.00 per month of the best all-in-one vitamins on the market. I figured that this would correct all the fast food that I was eating. It was a kind of "balancing" act I figured. Like buying a diet coke with a hamburger, or getting a salad…drenched with Thousand Island dressing, egg, chicken, bacon strips and maybe some buttered croutons. Besides, that's what the advertisements said could happen. I trusted the Ads.

I would be lying if I didn't tell you I noticed an increase in energy after taking about $1000.00 of vitamins. I decided the next step would be to add more vitamins to my "all-in-one" vitamin. I didn't like giving up that huge cupboard in my kitchen for vitamin storage and hauling around 15 bottles of vitamins everywhere I went. However, if I could keep eating the fast food, it was worth it. I liked the idea so much that I decided to open up a vitamin store and teach people this concept...How's that for a confessional?

I figured I could start showing people how to have a crutch and still eat the SAD diet (although, at the time I didn't see it as a crutch of course. I saw it as the answer). I didn't realize at the time that the all-in-one vitamin that I was taking was synthetic and made in a laboratory. It was the very same place that the medicine I used to take was being made! I also did not realize that doctors and scientists were deciding how much magnesium was needed to synthesize the calcium in my body. I trusted synthetic vitamins. Interestingly, I did notice that I was still getting colds and flu and my weight was still gaining on me. Off and on over those years I had now tried just about every diet that had been advertised to me. I was known as the good ol' "yoyo." One month I would be 30 pounds lighter and the next month, I would be 35 pounds heavier. I literally had to keep two sets of clothes for this way of life. I would gain weight until my large set of clothes was tight and then I would starve myself for a month and put on my skinnier clothes. As soon as I would go back to my SAD eating I would blow up and trump my "heavy" record in no time at all. This was my life.

I was losing the battle...

Eventually, I reached almost 60 pounds overweight (I was obese). My blood pressure was at about 210 over 110. My cholesterol was over 300. My triglycerides were over 600. Even my triceratops, my T-Rex and my gullibles were astronomical at one point, I think. Everything was wonky. When I went to sleep, I couldn't lay on my right side because of the chest pain I had when I laid down. I would have to turn over about every 30 minutes in the night because my acid reflux would get so bad. I would get winded simply walking up our stairs. My back hurt all the time, my knees were hurting. And now a new hurt had really taken first place: I had arthritis in both my thumbs and big toes. This was not fun. And yet, as I shared previously, it was the "best there was". I was living, sort of, with what I had been given. I was like many American people. I lingered more than lived.

I decided to try some of those super fruits being advertised. You know the ones that come in a quart bottle and cost 40 bucks. At the time I didn't know that they had been pasteurized and all the live enzymes were now dead in it and the sugar content was sky high in them. I trusted super fruits. I was determined not to go to the doctors and take meds for all these problems that were now popping up. After all, I was only 47. I didn't have a place to go. I finally didn't trust the doctors. I finally didn't trust the all-in-one vitamin. One night, sitting at my computer, the world started spinning on me. I was only 47 years old. This could not be happening to me. I was taking my crutch vitamins; I was eating a healthy SAD diet. And…I was rushed to the hospital that night. The doctors were able to get my blood pressure down some but said that I had to start on meds now to keep it down or I was a walking time bomb. I came home exhausted and confused. I didn't want to go back to all the meds again. I remembered how lousy I felt taking meds.

I was lying on the couch trying to process all this when my wife came up and handed me a Hallelujah Acres book and pleaded for me to read it. I thought it would maybe help get my mind off the terrible shape that I was in. I started reading it and noticed a few things that were interesting. They were not promoting new drugs. They were not promoting all-in-one vitamins. They were promoting scripture from the Bible of all things! They were promoting vegetables. Everyone knows that there is no money in promoting vegetables. What was their motive? Where is the catch? Were they "selling me God"? The more I read, the more I got interested in what my wife had told me to do for the past 10 years. I went to their website and started searching testimonies. I could not believe that just eating vegetables could help heal all these diseases. I read about people being healed of cancer. I read about people being healed of diabetes, lupus, fibromyalgia, colitis, crones, MS. I got excited when I read that even arthritis and heart disease and acid reflux responded to this lifestyle. I kept reading and searching and learning that our bodies were created to heal themselves if we would just put the correct nutrition in and get the toxins out. This sounded too easy. No doctors were needed to tell me what to take. I had to make a choice that night. Do I go the doctor way and go on all these meds or do I try this natural way and let my body heal itself? I chose the natural way. It would be plant based eating and cooking for me.

I think my wife must have thought that I had overdosed on meds because I went to the refrigerator and started tossing out all my cheese, milk, and butter. She really got scared when I went to the freezer and started throwing out my steaks, hot dogs, deer meat and pork. Although, later, needless to say, she was one happy camper that I had chosen this direction after all. My new direction was not without "issues"…

After about three days on this new lifestyle I felt worse than ever. My body broke out in hives, my head ached and I was exhausted. No one had mentioned the "detox" word. Once I started putting the nutrition in that my body needed, my body started to clean house. I was detoxing from all ports and no matter how pressed I am, I won't share with any great length, what ports those were. But then, another two days of this and things started looking up. I noticed that I was not tired as much. My head was clearing up. And the best thing (according to my wife) was that I had stopped snoring! I was drinking carrot juice and taking this yucky green drink and eating all these salads. I sure didn't like the taste of this new lifestyle, but I had to admit that I had not felt this good in years and I had only been going for a week.

My habits changed quite a bit. Every time I wanted to eat a piece of meat or cheese, I would think about the meds that I would need. I sure missed that good SAD food. I also noticed that my weight was dropping rapidly, my blood pressure had come down some and my chest pain had almost completely gone away. I started exercising by walking. At first it was a short distance only. I would get out of breath quickly, but I would continue for a little farther every time I went out. Before I knew it, I was walking a mile and not out of breath.

I dropped 20 pounds the first month. My skin tone had changed drastically. My blood pressure was down to normal without medications. Wow, did I feel dumb. I had been playing in the wrong game for decades and hurting the whole time. Now, after one month my body felt like a kid again. I want to be clear: I still didn't like the taste of the food. My wife had been begging to go to a Hallelujah Acre Lifestyle center and learn more about the do's and don'ts of this way of living. She also mentioned that they teach you how to cook great tasting plant based foods. All my life I loved cooking. I could make the best lasagna, steaks and Mexican food anywhere. That was a passion of mine. I started thinking to myself. Why not become the best "plant food" chef out there? That would be a good challenge to try, and I would sure enjoy the lifestyle more if I could have some better tasting foods.

We went to the Hallelujah Lifestyle center in Lake Lure, North Carolina run by Tim and Anita Koch. She had been a chef herself in New York for many years. There were about 10 people there that stayed at their center for five days. In that five days, they explained to us how we get our protein, calcium, vitamins, minerals all from eating plant based food. We had hands on cooking classes twice a day. We learned how to slice and dice. We learned how to make smoothies, juices and even decadent desserts. When we left there, we felt that we could live this way and really enjoy eating this way. By now, I felt like a 20 year old. I was 48 and jogging up hills that I would not even think of walking up 6 months prior.

My wife is a very patient lady. I think she had this planned from the start. She asked me if I might be interested in opening up a lifestyle center in Branson, MO. We could go to the Hallelujah Acres headquarters and get more training and then teach people how to get healthy and feel so much better. I agreed and off we went. We've not stopped learning to this day. It's great. We now have seen with our own eyes all these diseases disappear. We have witnessed so many people come through our Lifestyle center and see their life change in a matter of 5 days. We get letters and e-mails daily of people thanking us for teaching them how to live this way. We have letters from people that have gotten off 8 medications that they had been on for years. Others have lost more than 100 pounds. I have lost more than 50 pounds myself. I have not weighed this little since high school. Yes, I had to go and buy all new cloths, so that hurt my frugal thinking for a while. The most common comment that we got was "I can't believe that this food tastes so good and it can be good for you". You should open up a restaurant. We have thought about that idea but we would have to give up our lifestyle center if we did.

I decided to do the first best thing and that is write a cook book. I have been asked hundreds of times to write a cook book. I knew that there were thousands of cook books on the market and I did not want to be a dust collector on somebody's kitchen counter. I have put a lot of thought into this and tried to come up with a happy medium. I would write a cook book and teach at the same time. I would let people know why they should eat that stalk of celery or why they should add spinach to their smoothie (yes, I am serious). I would show them how to mix and match vegetable to make even a SAD eater love their food. I was asked if there was a cook book out there that had a plan for the week or month of what to buy, what to cook. I decided to add all these "ingredients" to this cook book.

So get ready for an adventure. As I said earlier, this isn't a one-step plan. This is a lifestyle plan...comprehensive in every way. I will show you how to prepare incredible meals that you can serve to your animal eating friends and they won't even miss the meatless dishes. I will give you recipes that are wonderful tasting and at the same time give you an alternate way of preparing it for someone dealing with disease. You can feel good about what you are eating and know that you are putting in the proper nutrition to let your body heal itself of all these diseases. I have even added a section showing you the advantages of eating certain vegetables for certain issues. I even added a dessert section. My hope is to give you a cook book where you can open to any page and know that you are about to eat the healthiest way possible, as well as the "best tasting" way possible. Enjoy...

For additional teaching and recipes, please visit our website and blog at Godsfoodnow.com

Getting Started

So the big question is: How exactly do YOU begin a new way of eating....a new lifestyle? How do you take your own story of how unhealthy or healthy you are and become an expert at eating right? I've shared my story – for better or worse – but that doesn't really get you any closer to getting healthy other than letting you know that you are not alone, right? But that IS the first step of getting healthy, believe it or not! You see, by understanding that there is an entire nation that has fallen into a sort of "sleep" about health and eating the best way possible, we kind of share a similar story. We all, at one point or another have been duped by a system, both in medicine and health ideas we've been sold. We've been told time and time again a series of myths about eating. The frequency by which we are told these myths is so rapid that we are bound to believe it. How could we not, right? It's like the old marketing adage, familiarity equals credibility. The more you are exposed to something as the truth the more you'll begin to believe it's so. It's as though our psychological belief system is based upon a "general consensus" about facts. If enough people support it, and it's seen by many people, well then it must be true. But, that is exactly the wrong way to think about the truth.

Truth isn't about consensus. It's about deliberate, diligent, and specific actions to discover, explore and understand what really is happening in order to create a legitimate belief with interconnected rules of order. That doesn't mean you have to distrust everything until you are happy it's true. The fact is you won't necessarily understand how everything works. So I want to qualify my statement by saying some truths are "self-evident" because of the tested nature of them. In other words, you may believe you can fly. But go ahead and jump off a roof and you'll soon discover that your exploration should have relied on other knowledge than your own to baseline your truth. What I am talking about here is the ability to test some truths so that you don't just accept it wholesale. Going back to the truth that you'll likely end up very hurt (if not worse) should you jump off a rooftop, it would be safe to say that you simply have to look at examples of others to know they got hurt...leading to a reasonable conclusion that you too would get hurt. There may be stand out cases where someone survived without injury...but those are exceptions rather than rules that are being developed. If we were to shift over to the idea of health and eating, we could extrapolate similar truths about some health concepts while others would begin to shake you up a bit.

Let's look at an example of a health "truth" to give you some clarity on what I mean. Many years ago there was a research study done on the correlation between heart attacks and drinking coffee. It turns out, after surveying, following and researching the target group (In this case, coffee drinkers), that there was an increased risk of heart attack. It was troubling for many people when the research was published. The implication was massive. The coffee industry would have to contend with the fact that their beverage was causing people to die from heart attacks! And then, a while later, more in-depth analysis was done on the "truth" that coffee was causing these problems. Eventually, it was vetted out that there was a miscalculation of sorts on the study. You see, it became clear after more diligence that the coffee drinkers that were studied also had a penchant for smoking. Every time they went out for a cup of coffee they also typically lit up a cigarette. It turns out that it wasn't the coffee that was causing heart attack issues…it was the smoking that accompanied the coffee drinking. Another study revealed that coffee by itself did nothing to increase any risk of heart problems. In fact, recently a study suggested that drinking coffee in the right amounts even lowered the risk of heart disease by up to 34% in women and 44% in men. How's that for a flip flop in "truths"?

So what are we supposed to believe? If one study can say one thing and another say something completely different, who are we to believe? And, furthermore, why not simply vacillate with the research? There's no point in waiting things out is there?

The honest answer is yes and no. We are all individuals. As such we have to see how our body responds to certain things. I wouldn't advise a "one-size-fits-all" approach to anything, especially health. Rather, I think we have to try to see what works for us. Look at the truths, discover alternatives and understand that statistics are just that. They are based on an average over all. You may be the exception. Or you may have a particular food allergy that would keep you from some foods that help many others. The key is to look at what others have done, study the options for you and then make a decision about the best possible track. Read about trusted methods, but don't just take the words of "experts" on it. Read up on it, even this recipe/cookbook. Make sure what I'm writing here isn't your only option. While it's a great option, it may not be for everyone. I do share valuable strategies that have been proven and I have seen as a first hand witness to be effective. But results vary. You are unique and as such you have to make sure that your approach is tied to you, not just what everyone else is saying.

Let's go one final time to the rooftop example. You can believe you can fly. You can believe you can't fly. You can read about others who've tried and failed and even those miraculous attempts where the survivors walked away unharmed. I advocate looking at all the options before trying the next step up there because honestly, the repercussions of your decisions will impact you (pun not intended) for years to come. They might even impact you for the rest of your life. So, what are you going to do to get started? Are you going to walk, run or fly off that roof? Or are you going to look at your options and discover some truths I personally have explored that God willing, will also impact you in a very personal, purposeful and healthy way? If you chose the second option, read on as I get down to the basics of preparing for a new life of health and feeling better than you can imagine. And remember, what I write here isn't just a research paper, or a study. It's a long term commitment to finding the best foods, cooking and ways to better health. Not magic pills…just honest to goodness advice, food and good eating!

You are going to need a blender and a food processor of some kind. There is simply no way around it. If you have these items, great! If not - I have found several good places to shop for appliances and food items. I have listed them on my website: www.Godsfoodnow.com. This site will give you ideas of where to get your organic foods, nuts, beans and hard to get items. It has specials every month on appliances that will make your life much easier.

Remember, these are items that are going to make your life a lot easier, so don't go out and buy the cheapest brand. Make sure what you get performs well and is durable. I would recommend a 9 – 12 cup food processor for a family of 4 or larger. This machine will shave hours a week off your time.

While there are many options and many costs available, basically only two blenders are worth your money and time, in my opinion. The

Powermill and the Vitamix are amazing blenders. These two blenders are strong enough to make hummus or frozen smoothies. The Powermill is about half the price of the Vita Mix and just as good. Do, if you're on a budget, go for the Powermill.

With the food processor and the blender you can more than equip your kitchen into a user friendly environment for plant based cooking. Other items to buy in the future would include a food dehydrator to create some wonderful snacks and foods for storage. You can also use it to gently heat food which keeps the enzymes alive if you do not take it to hot. Another item to have is a pressure cooker. Yes, I know your grandmother blew up her kitchen with this appliance. Pressure cookers like many kitchen appliances have come a long way though. They are safer today and make cooking so much easier. When buying a pressure cooker, buy only stainless steel. Do not buy the aluminum models because it could possibly leach metals into your body via the foods you cook.

Once you have the equipment that you will need, it is time to clean house! If you leave all the goodies and snacks and meats and cheeses laying around, it will be very hard to not fall off the wagon and cave into snacking on these items again. Yes, they cost money at one time, but you need to realize that these foods are what got you into the poor health or lack of energy or overweight place to begin with. Give them away or throw them away; if you don't they'll have a tendency to keep showing up somehow. Even if you are planning on transitioning slowly into this lifestyle, it is recommended to get rid of all junk food immediately. If you are going to splurge one day, then go buy only enough for that one time and give the rest away. I am so adamant about this point I want you to do one thing for me right now. Put the book down, go to your kitchen, grab a trash bag and dump every single junk food package, bag or container away. Return when you're done. Do it. Go on…I'll be here waiting.

Transitioning to a healthier lifestyle

So here is secret number two in our journey: Most people go about transitioning to a better lifestyle of eating and health in the wrong way. They will eat 70% well, and have just a little "bad food" every single day. Majority wins, right? If you're doing mostly "good" that's better than doing mostly "bad". It's the old "diet coke and a hamburger" routine again.

The main problem with this technique of eating well is that you never get to feel the feeling of good health because your body always has some bad food running through it. The transition from a bad diet to a good one never gets entirely done. Instead of transitioning without ever transitioning completely, I recommend that you commit to going several days without eating any bad food. It's tough. And it'll require endurance and a strong will. But it can be done. And you'll be amazed at how well it will work. Rather than have a little bad food every day, limit it to specific days where "bad food" is allowed. But don't eat poorly outside that day...and eventually reduce those allowed bad days.

 Pick a day a week to begin where you'll *eliminate "bad food" entirely.* What you don't want to do is have just a little piece of chocolate here, or a little slice of cheese there, each day. That keeps your body from being able to run clean and start fixing the problems it has. Have a "pig out" day if you need to. Get it all out of your system in one day and then get back on track. This way your body can heal.

Set a goal. Maybe during month one, allow yourself a pig out day on the weekends. Then month two, extend it to only two days a month for "bad food". Eventually you will find that you are feeling so good eating healthy that you really don't want to pig out as much. It becomes less and less alluring to eat poorly or eat too much. It becomes like your body is having a food hangover. If you are not fighting any serious disease your body can handle a few bad food days a month.

What you'll find during this correct transition is that It's such a wonderful feeling to start getting healthy again. It is amazing and revelatory to discover how much you are missing by eating the junk foods from before. All of a sudden you start having more energy. Your clarity of mind comes back. Those little aches and pains are no longer hanging around. You forget what a headache or allergy feels like. It is so worth eating good food. But remember: this is not like a drug that you take and 20 minutes later you feel different. Instead, your body is healing itself slowly. It took a long time to get you in the shape you are in today. Don't expect to have that euphoria back overnight. Hang in there and it will pay big dividends. I have found in our center that people staying on the lifestyle start feeling better by day four. From there it just keeps getting better and better every day.

Don't be surprised that you feel worse before you feel better though. As soon as you start putting the good fuel only in your body, your body is going to want to get busy fixing all the problems. Many people will feel cold or flu-like symptoms on day two and three. This is a good thing. It is your body detoxifying and getting rid of all the bad stuff. By day four you will start turning the corner and wow what a great feeling it is.

Be sure to start a journal. I encourage you to write down on a piece of paper all your aches and pains and problems. Write down things like how often you have a head ache, allergies, snoring (yes, you will find that most of your snoring will go away on day four), brittle finger nails, nail biting, sore muscles, sore joints acne, body odor, bad breath. Then take that journal list back out in one month and review all the issues that no longer exist. You will be amazed at your discovery! Another big plus by eating this way is getting off all those medications. Remember my story? My blood pressure was 210 over 110 when I started on this lifestyle. It now averages 125 over 70 without medication. Almost every type two diabetic that has followed this lifestyle has been able to get completely off medication. The list goes on and on.

We have many people get off more than 8 medications in a very short period of time. They can't believe how much better they feel not taking all those meds. It is worth the change. Stick with it for a month before you make any decisions on how you will eat the rest of your life. Give yourself a sort of trial run. Remember the key is eat healthy most of the time, not just some of the time. The principle we have to understand is that we have to change our mind set to the *opposite* of what it has been. We need to think about keeping good food as the norm and bad food as a rare "treat". Soon, you'll regard that "treat' as something entirely different.

The "whys" and "why nots" of plant based eating

Believe it or not, in Genesis 1:29, God gives man his first menu of food to eat. God told man that any seed bearing plant and any fruit bearing tree shall be your meat. This was God's best for us. He didn't say eat vitamins. He didn't say use a supplement. He didn't even say eat mostly fast food or frozen foods. You'll even notice that no disease is mentioned in scripture until meat is introduced in the Bible. Don't get me wrong. I do not state that to suggest it is a sin to eat meat or fish at all. However; I do want to point out that animal products have changed dramatically since God created them.

Scripture does tell us how to eat meat, interestingly enough. There are guidelines to preparation of the meat by bleeding it a certain way. We are told not to eat the fat. In today's meat there are tons of hormones and vaccines pumped into the cattle. The average cow is now approaching 30 percent fat content due to a desire to provide more "tasty" meat. Because of that, though, we can no longer remove the fat as we are instructed to in Scripture. The fat is now infused throughout the entire meat cut. Even with the wonderful fish of the sea we are finding so many pollutants that they are likely unfit to eat. Mercury levels are so high that sometimes the fish is even dangerous to eat. It is sad that our waters and seas are so polluted that we cannot eat what swims in it.

Think about this for a moment: have you noticed that our kids are now hitting puberty some three and four years earlier? The reason lies partly in all the hormones stored in our foods. Young girls are now marrying at 9 and 10 years old. And they experience menstruation sometimes even younger. Young boys are getting facial hair at 11 and 12 years old. With all the hormones in the chicken and beef that pass into our bodies we are having a chemical reaction that is changing who we are and how we grow! Man has taken what God created as good and turned it into bad. It is important that we get this concept in our thinking.

The fact of the matter is that when we ingest animal product it does interesting things to our blood. About 3 years ago I went to a doctor and had my blood drawn and put under a microscope to be viewed live. It was very interesting to see the blood cells moving around in the plasma. They were all separated and zipping around in the plasma doing their job. I then went and ate a piece of cheese pizza I waited about an hour. I returned to the doctor and had my blood drawn again. What a difference. Now my cells were all clumped together and moving slowly around. You could actually see fat floating in the plasma. One of the major jobs of the red blood cells is to deliver oxygen and nutrition to your body. If your cells are clumped together, there is no way that they can deliver the oxygen and nutrition your body needs effectively. The reason is because animal fat does not melt at body temperature. As a comparison, all plant based fats do melt below body temperature. Clearly now, you can see why people start seeing dramatic physical changes in their body soon after eliminating the animal products from their diet.

How to Get Fat the Easy Way

Obesity is easy to achieve when eating the Standard American Diet. We call this diet the S.A.D. Diet. When you look at the calorie density of animal product versus plant based product, it is typically a huge difference. For instance, if you were to steam some broccoli and cauliflower and make a baked potato verses making a cooked lasagna with a side of white bread sticks covered in oil or butter, you would be eating three or four times the calories in one sitting. Do this at every meal and it is easy to understand why we are such an obese nation. Ready for this? When eating a plant based diet, you don't have to count calories. It's actually difficult to eat too much food when you eat a plant based menu.

Most all of your processed foods found in grocery stores or a big box stores have many chemicals for preserving and for adding flavors. One of the worst is MSG. This terrible chemical is used in many of our foods today and it is called so many different names that it is difficult to keep up with which word they are currently using for this chemical. MSG kills brain cells at such a rapid rate it's boggling. It also stimulates our taste buds to eat more of this artificial food that has been laced with it. And yet, while we eat so much of it, we are unaware of the harm that it's causing us. Basically, (and I know this may be hard for you) I would highly recommend staying away from all processed foods if you are able to. They have to add so many chemicals and preservatives in order to meet FDA rules and standards. Any time you put chemicals like MSG and others in your system, it takes days to get it out…and that is if your body is in decent shape. Think of how long it takes if you're not in tip top shape.

On the other hand, when you choose to put nothing but fruits and vegetables into your system, your body starts cleansing and detoxifying immediately. When you choose to use this energy source your body knows exactly what to do with it. Anytime you eat raw vegetables, it is even better because all the enzymes are still attached to the food. These enzymes are like an owner's manual. They tell your body how to utilize the food and send it to the proper places. Importantly, they also tell your body not to store it as fat either. A good habit to get in is to always eat your raw salad or foods first. This sets up your system to accept food and realize that it is a good thing coming in rather than a possible toxin or poison.

I would like to touch on the common myth of protein deficiency when eating a plant based diet. The fact is there is a lot of protein in vegetables. For a clear example of how much protein there is in plants and veggies look at the cows and horses in the field. Where did they get their protein? Not from eating other cows. The protein found in vegetables is a much better protein for humans than that found in animal product because plant based protein is not a complete protein. What this means is that it doesn't go too rapidly into our system. When a protein goes into our system too fast it generates issues. Instead, plant-based proteins are stored and when the body is in need of a certain amino acid or protein, it can draw on that particular protein and use only what is needed.

Dr. T. Colin Campbell did a multi-year study in China and found that most diseases are not present or even known in the areas where animal product was not consumed. He also noted that there was little or no osteoporosis, heart disease, cancer, lupus or high blood pressure in plant-based eating villages. The villages made for a perfect study because the village had eaten the same diet for all its existence – with no influence of animal product consumption. The even more interesting thing in his decades long study was that when the team of researches came to villages where animal product and higher protein consumptions were found, then also all the western diseases were found. Dr. Campbell's team spent many hours studying the involvement of protein and cancer. They found that in rats they could turn on and turn off cancer cells just by adjusting the amount of protein in their diets. We Americans have been told that we have to have all these grams of protein to sustain a healthy body. I am sorry to tell you this is a great myth...one that is hurting you. Most information about eating more meat is coming directly from the beef industry. It's an industry that is powerful, global and lobbies constantly, while spending too much money promoting the faulty link between eating meat and gaining health.

Think about it. Have you ever thought about who dictates what we eat? We think we are in charge of our decisions, but are we really? Who makes your kid's school lunch menus? Did you know there is a ton of red tape to get schools to *not serve* your child a carton of milk? As a parent, you have to submit a ton of paper work, pleading with them, convincing them that you do not want your child to drink milk. Why? For starters, it's the dairy industry that dictates what your child eats and drinks at school. Did you know that government subsidizes meat and dairy specifically? What if you had to pay the real price for this type of food? You would see a lot more and more healthy people out there for one thing. But for another, you'd see that we have these multi-billion dollar industries working ever so hard to train your child and your family to eat more meat, drink more milk and get hooked on a diet that doesn't serve you but serves their pocket books. And the price you pay is greater than the subsidized industry monies…you pay weight, your health and with your life.

Got Strong Bones?

I want to touch on calcium deficiency for a moment. It is interesting that the US has one of the highest osteoporosis rates in the world. Why would that be? We have the best doctors; we have the best medicine; we have all the tools necessary to overcome so much, and we all drink milk like we're told. Yet here we stand as a country of sickly boned people. Well, did you know that there are studies that show that the consumption of milk will actually *reduce your calcium levels*? Don't just believe me. Go out there and read the studies and research that the Dairy industry doesn't want you to read. You see, milk is an animal product. Any time we put animal product in our body, we are creating an acid environment. Any time we have an acid environment we have to counteract it with an alkaline like calcium. Our diets are so heavy laden with meats and dairy and processed foods that are all very acidic in nature. Plainly put – it takes a serious toll on our bodies as we continue eating this way. The way to stop osteoporosis is not adding calcium to our diets as suggested (which is very hard to absorb) but to stop putting so much acid in our bodies to begin with.

Eating plant-based foods and cooking with them isn't a new idea but it's a life-saving one. So many people think that eating vegetables and fruits, etc., is boring and won't feed their body correctly. But (SAD)ly they are living a lie. It is the meat and processed foods that are creating most of the health issues to begin with. What do you do when you have a problem? You don't just bandage it up you remove the source of the problem. By removing meats from your diet (even mostly) you will see a new you emerge. That new you will weigh less, have better health and less disease. The principle to remember is that switching to a plant based diet as opposed to the Standard American Diet will help you gain health in a slowly withering culture. Stop accepting the lies and start living in health.

Food items to buy

To start living that life of health you desire you'll need some special food items that are used in plant based eating. I would recommend going to your local health food store and getting these items to start. You can also go to my website and I have posted some online stores that are very cheap and very good. They will drop ship directly to your house. You typically have to buy a larger quantity but the price difference makes it well worth it. As a note when shopping, when I'm buying bulk, I always store my excess nuts and grains in my freezer to keep them fresh. You may want to do the same. In the following sections I more fully explain how to buy for long periods of time rather than one day at a time.

Here is a list of needed items:

Nutritional Yeast Flakes – This is non-active yeast. It will not cause any yeast or Candida issues like brewer's yeast can. It is also very high in B vitamins. This is what we use to get a cheesy flavor in many recipes. Start with 1lb.

Raw sunflower seeds – This is a great way to get protein. Raw sunflower seeds are almost one third protein. You can get your daily protein needs met by eating sunflower seeds. Start with at least 3lbs.

Raw cashews - This nut is used in desserts and salad dressings. You can buy small pieces instead of whole cashews because you will be chopping or blending them anyway. Start with at least 3lbs.

Raw Walnuts - Walnuts are one of the best nuts to eat. They are very high in Omega 3. Start with 3 LBS.

Raw Almonds - Almonds are used in many of the desserts and are also a good snack when you need a fix. Start with 3lbs.

Oatmeal – I would recommend buying organic oatmeal if you can. My website has a source for it. Oatmeal is a good filler when you are craving junk food.

Wheat Germ – This is used in my veggie burger and is packed with nutrition. Start with 1lb.

Braggs Liquid Aminos – You can also use Tamari or Nama Shoyu. All 3 of these can be substituted for each other. Start with 1 Quart. Vegenaise – This is a healthy (as healthy as possible) Mayonnaise. Only buy the grape seed oil version. I do not believe in using Canola oil. You should read how Canola oil was created and you might rapidly follow suit. Start with 1 quart.

Brown Rice – Basmati brown rice is excellent. Never use white rice. All the good has been taken out of it and the white rice will just plug up your digestive system and keep it from working properly. Think whole grain from this day forward for any breads, pasta or rices. The processed white foods cause so many problems in your body.
Wild rice – This is a good rice to mix with brown rice dishes. You don't have to use much to add lots of color and flavor.

Rice pasta – A good substitute is rice pasta. You can also use whole wheat pasta. If you do, make sure it is not "enriched". That means that it is not a whole grain and they have added chemicals back to it, maybe even MSG.

Agave Nectar – Make sure you buy raw agave nectar.

Honey - Make sure you buy raw honey. It is best if you can find a local honey. It is said to help with allergies if you use local honey because the bee's have gone and grabbed pollen from these weeds and put it in the honey. Then your body will slowly build a defense against these allergies in the honey.

Coconut oil - This is one of the better oils for you. It can also take higher heats and does not break down as fast when using in cooking.

Coconut flakes - This is used in desserts and you can also make coconut water with it much cheaper than buying coconut water. Just mix ½ cup flakes with 1 cup water and blend well.

Sea Salt - Throw away all your regular salts. They are terrible for you. You can use most any sea salt and be safe.

Flax seed - This is a great way to get omega 3. It is also used as a thickener for many recipes. Seasonings to buy:

Here are some of the more frequently used seasonings to help you get started on the right track. You are likely familiar with most if not all of them. Used in the right combinations they make for some amazing dishes. But more of that in the recipe section!

Basil
Oregano
Garlic powder
Onion powder
Coriander
Cumin
Dill weed
Soy hickory flavoring.

Three Days at a Time

One of the challenges to eating in our new health lifestyle is that you will be eating lots of good food. So in order to prep ahead of time, rather than "make as you go" and therefore, take perhaps too much time per day, I've included a way to shop for eating three days at a time. Over the next couple pages you'll find a comprehensive list of the prep foods you'll need to buy for making your meals three days at a time. Make sure you put this on your grocery list as you get ready to realize some terrific health benefits.

Shopping List – Days 1 through 3

Broccoli	7 heads
Cabbage-white	1 head
Green Onions	1 bunch
Lemons	7
Avocados	4
Potatoes	4 LG
Corn	6 Ears
Red Bell Peppers	3
Celery	1 bunch
Kale	3 bunches
Cilantro	1 bunch
Frozen Peas	1 bag
Tomatoes	2
Onions	2
Sweet Potatoes	2
Sundried Tomatoes	1 jar
Portabella	1 flat
Carrots	1 LB
Cauliflower	1 head
Oranges	7
Strawberries	1 pint
Blueberries	1 Quart
Limes	4
Frozen Raspberries	1 bag
Bananas	22

Ripen your bananas until they have brown freckles, then peel and freeze in Zip-lock baggies for smoothies later on.

Shopping List – Days 4 through 7

Bananas	20	peel & freeze
pineapple	1	
pears	3	
apples	4	
cantalope	1	
melon	1	
blueberries	3 pints	
raspberries-frozen	2 pints	
strawberries	1 quart	
Mangos	2	
Sweet potato	4	
pecans	1 sm bag	
cucumber	8	
Roma tomatoes	17	
avocado	4	
Lemons	4	
red bell pepper	6	
sweet onion	4	
green olives	1 jar	
sliced mushrooms	1 pint	
yellow bell pepper	4	

Spinach	2 LB
broccoli	1
zucchini	4
yellow squash	1
tomatoes - diced 28oz can	1
romaine lettuce	3 heads
black olives	1 jar
dill weed	1 pkt
celery	1 bunch
green onions	1 bunch
limes	6
Wheat Germ	1 LB
mushrooms	1 pint
parsley	1 bunch
sun dried tomatoes	1 jar
sliced mushrooms	1 pint
can green chilies	1
refried beans	1 lg can
almonds	2 cups
cashews	3 cups
dates	1 cup
honey	1 cup

7 Day Meal Plan

Day 1

Breakfast: Oatmeal with Raisins and Walnuts (pg 264)

Smoothie: In a blender add, 1 peeled orange, 4 frozen bananas, juice from 1 lime, 1 pint strawberries, 1 cup water. Blend well and serve.

Lunch: Broccoli/Cabbage and avocado slices. You can add some whole grain crackers if you wish. Use sparingly.

*Try to avoid drinking liquids with your meals. This has a tendency to dilute the stomach acids

Dinner: Cheesy Baked Potatoes (pg 221) and Sweet Corn Salad (pg 140)

*When at all possible, you will want to go for a walk after each meal. Your body will love you for it and you will love your body after it.

Day 2

Breakfast: Bananas, apples and blueberries

*Try to eat all the different fruits. This is important in order to get all the different nutrients from the different fruits and vegetables.

Smoothie: In a blender add, 1 peeled orange, 4 frozen bananas, juice from one lime, 1 pint blueberries, 1 cup water. Blend well and serve.

Lunch: Broccoli Pea Salad (pg 148) and sliced tomatoes. You may add whole grain crackers. Use sparingly.

Dinner: Stuffed Bell Peppers (pg 197) and Caesar Salad

Day 3

Breakfast: Oatmeal, walnuts and apples.

Smoothie: In a blender add, 1 peeled orange, 4 frozen bananas, juice from 1 lime, 1 pint of raspberries, 1 cup water. Blend well and serve.

Lunch: Rainbow Salad (pg 153) with Sweet Onion Salad Dressing (pg 266) and Green Onion Hummus (pg 115).

Dinner: Beaf Strogonaff (pg 185) and Kale Salad (pg 157)

*Use Tinkyada rice noodles, they cook really easily. When you get them to the desired texture, run cool water over them so they stop cooking. When making the salad, be sure to squeeze/massage the kale for at least 2 minutes.

Day 4

Breakfast: Bananas, apples and blueberries

Smoothie: In a blender add, 1 peeled orange, 4 frozen bananas, juice from one lime, ½ pineapple, 2 mangos peeled, 1 cup water. Blend well and serve. Add some coconut flakes for that Piña Colada taste if you like.

Lunch: Zucchini Salad (pg 174) and celery sticks

Dinner: Tuscan Pasta (pg 205) and Sweet Potato Salad (pg 172)

*Use Tinkyada rice noodles for the pasta

Day 5

Breakfast: Oatmeal, walnuts and raisins

*Add a small amount of honey or Agave nectar to sweeten. Another healthy tip is to grind up 1 Tbsp of flax seed and add to oatmeal.

Smoothie: In a blender add, 1 peeled orange, 4 frozen bananas, juice from 1 lime, 1 handful each of blueberries, raspberries and strawberries, 1 cup water. Blend well and serve.

Lunch: Spinach Pear Salad (pg 170) with Tomato Pesto Hummus (pg 108)

Dinner: Coconut Vegetables (pg 202) with House Salad (pg 179) and Thousand Island Dressing (pg 256).

Day 6

Breakfast: Cantaloupe and Melon. Cube melons and serve.

*There is an old saying, Eat melons alone or leave melons alone. Melons digest very fast and if added with other foods, it has a tendency to ferment the other food. Remember "Melons Alone."

Smoothie: In a blender add, 1 peeled orange, 4 frozen bananas, juice from 1 lime, 1 handful each of blueberries, strawberries and raspberries, 1 cup of water. Blend well and serve.

Lunch: Cucumber Dill Salad (pg 121) and Gazpacho Soup (pg 138)

Dinner: Veggie Burgers (pg 192) and Avocado Salad (pg 135)

*Don't get worried when you see the veggie burger recipe with all the ingredients. Use your food processor and mince all ingredients. It is very fast. One hint: process ingredients separately. Don't worry about cleaning the processor between vegetables because you are mixing them all together anyway. This will make extra burgers. They are wonderful as a snack or freeze them for another meal. They are great to add to your spaghetti also.

Day 7

Breakfast: Oatmeal, walnuts and apples

Smoothie: In a blender add, 1 peeled orange, 4 frozen bananas, juice from 1 lime, 1 handful each of blueberries, raspberries and strawberries, 1 cup water. Blend well and serve.

Lunch: Spinach Almond Salad (pg 128) and Creamy Tomato Soup (pg 146)

Dinner: Fajitas (pg 209) and Refried Beans (pg 255) and Cheese Cake (pg 246)

*One of my favorites. You can add a few drops of liquid smoke to get that meaty flavor going. Add whatever vegetable that you love. The all go well in this dish. I will slice carrots and sauté them also. Add some yellow and green bell peppers or even some pineapple chunks if you like sweets.

*Wait until you try this cheesecake. It is the best of the best. You need to make this at least 4 hours prior to serving and better if you can make it the day before. Put it in the freezer and let it set up for hours. Remove about 30 minutes prior to serving. Add the topping just before serving. You can also change the flavor by using different toppings. Make a tasty carob/agave/vanilla topping for a change. Use ½ cup carob, ½ cup agave and 1 tsp vanilla. Blend and pour over

cheesecake or serve it on the side.

Recipes for feeling better today

Now it's time to get to the good stuff! In this section you'll get my cookbook recipes and helpful tips for better health. To be as clear as possible, I've broken the sections into specific meals and snack times to better help you understand the times and foods you're eating. So, you'll find sections for appetizers, soups and salads, main dishes, breads and rolls, desserts and miscellaneous foods. Each recipe in this cookbook is designed to give you optimum flavor and pick me up, while working long term to get your body more healthy. Enjoy…

APPETIZERS

What kind of nuts should I eat?

Always eat raw nuts. The nuts in a can are all roasted. Stay away from these. They will get you fat and they have bad oil after roasting. The best nut to eat is the Walnut. It has the best Omega 3 to Omega 6 ratio at about a 4-1 ratio. Other nuts have much higher ratios of omega 6. You want to try and get more Omega 3 in your diet. A great way to do that is with ground flax seed.

Tomato Pesto Hummus

- 1 large sweet potato
- 3 cloves garlic
- 1/3 cup water
- 1 cup raw sunflower seeds
- 1/4 fresh lemon juice
- 1/2 cup sun dried tomatoes

Place sun dried tomatoes in 1/3 water for 20

minutes. Add water and tomatoes and all

ingredients in blender and blend very well.

How to keep your Cilantro and Parsley fresh

When you buy Parsley or Cilantro, take the bunch and wrap the leaves in a paper towel and then put them in a plastic baggie with the stems hanging out. Keep them in your veggie drawer for more than a week and still have crisp leaves.

Almond Nut Spread

- 2 cups Almonds - soaked for 1 hour
- 1 cup Sunflower seeds soaked for 1 hour
- 2 Carrots - minced
- 3 stalks Celery - minced
- 1 Red Bell pepper - diced small
- 1/2 medium Sweet Onion - diced small
- 1 tablespoon onion powder
- 1 tablespoon Garlic powder
- 2 teaspoons Sea salt
- 3 tablespoons Fresh Lemon juice
- 1 tablespoon Honey
- 1/4 teaspoon Cayenne Pepper

Put almonds, sunflower seeds, lemon juice, garlic powder, onion powder, cayenne pepper, honey and sea salt into blender and blend well. Remove from blender and mix in all remaining diced ingredients. Serve over healthy crackers or toasted bread or celery sticks

Chipotle Hummus

- 3 cloves Garlic
- 2 cups Sunflower Seeds - raw
- 1/2 cup Fresh Lemon juice
- 1/4 cup Olive Oil
- 1/2 teaspoon Cumin
- 2 cups Sweet Potato
- 1/2 cup Tahini
- 1/2 cup Water
- 1 teaspoon Sea salt
- 1/2 teaspoon Tumeric
- 1/4 cup Chipotle Peppers

Soak sunflower seeds in water for 30 minutes and drain. Peel sweet potatoes and cube. Add all ingredients to blender and blend for several minutes until hummus is creamy and smooth. You can substitute roasted bell pepper for the chipotle if you do not want a spicy hummus. Serve with chips or crackers or sliced vegetables.

Where is the best place to buy produce?

I love the farmers markets. Here you have people that are passionate about what they do. They take pride in their work. They know how to work their fields of crops and when to pick at the peak freshness. You can ask them questions and they will help you. They have recipes to share and tricks on growing your own. If you go near the end of the day, you might even get some free veggies. When you are buying from a major store, they have to pick the produce days and sometimes weeks before peak freshness. You lose a bunch of nutrients when they do this. It is still better to buy from a major store than not eat at all. Do not use that as an excuse to go buy a Big Mac.

If you happen to have a www.Freggies.com location near you then you are in luck!

Green Onion Hummus

- 3 cloves Garlic
- 2 cups Sunflower Seeds - raw
- 1/2 cup Fresh Lemon juice
- 1/4 cup Olive Oil
- 1/2 teaspoon Cumin
- 1/2 teaspoon Tumeric
- 2 cups Sweet Potato
- 1/2 cup Tahini
- 1/2 cup Water
- 1 teaspoon Sea salt
- 5 Green Onions

Add all ingredients into a strong blender and blend very well. For additional flavors you can mince red bell pepper into the hummus..

I want to build muscle. How can I do that?

Many people think that eating a plant based diet low in protein will keep you from gaining muscle mass. The founder of Hallelujah Acres, Rev. George Malkmus at the young age of 70 plus decided to build muscle. This man has not eaten a piece of animal flesh or dairy in over 30 years. In less than a year, he added 2" of muscle to his biceps and triceps. Remember this man is over 70 years of age. There are many great nuts and vegetables that are high in protein values. One great seed is sunflower seeds. They are 33% protein. In 1 cup of sunflower seeds, you will get more than 30 grams of protein. For a growing boy, it is found that 10% of protein is sufficient. I would recommend making some of my hummus recipes. These recipes are packed with protein.

SOUPS & SALADS

How to peel an onion

Rumor has it that if you put the onion in the refrigerator for 30 minutes prior to peeling that you will not get teary eyes. Another wives tale has you cut out the root part of the onion. One of the more reliable methods we've seen is to hold a piece of bread on your mouth. But essentially, what you're trying to do is keep the juice from the onion from squirting in your eyes – which is what actually causes the onion peeling tearing up mess to happen in the first place.

Spanish Broccoli

- 3 cups broccoli
- 1/2 cup Toasted Almonds
- 1 Jalapeno
- 2 cloves Garlic
- 2 tablespoons Olive Oil
- 1/4 teaspoon Sea Salt
- 1/4 cup Cashews or Pine nuts
- 1/2 Avocado

Process Broccoli stems only in food processor using the S blade until stems are minced. Process broccoli tops in food processor until tops are about 1/4" in size. Take remaining ingredients except almonds and put in blender and blend until smooth. Mix dressing on broccoli and add toasted almonds and serve.

What is my ideal weight?

We are so focused on how much we weigh that we forget one easy method to determine our ideal weight. It is as simple as looking in the mirror. We are all made different and for us to use a predetermined weight does not make sense. Throw the scale away. Take a picture of you and post it on your mirror. Now start exercising and eating right and watch your body transform. You might actually gain weight as your body becomes full of muscle instead of the layers of fat. Muscle weighs almost 3 times that of fat for the same amount of volume. In other words, you can reduce your waist by several inches and gain weight. If you do, be happy because now muscle needs energy which burns calories. It is a great cycle to get into. As you add muscle and get in shape, your body needs more calories so it will have to burn more fat to maintain energy, now more rapidly converting your body to look better. Do not compare yourself to some overweight friend. Be honest with yourself. Do you still have a roll of fat on your waistline? Do your thighs jiggle? How about that behind? Does it look like it did in high school? This is the way to determine how much you should weigh. Let the mirror be the judge.

Cucumber Dill Salad

- 1 cup Cashews - soaked in water for 1 hour
- 1 cup Pine nuts - soaked in water for 1 hour
- 1/2 cup water
- 1/4 Fresh Lemon juice
- 1 teaspoon Sea salt
- 4 cloves Garlic
- 1 cup Fresh Dill or 2 Tbsp dry Dill Weed

Soak nuts for 1 hour and drain well. In a blender mix nuts, garlic, salt, lemon juice and water. Blend until creamy. Dice cucumbers into 1/2" cubes. Pat cucumbers dry with towel. Add all ingredients together and serve.

Is it better to eat raw or cooked vegetables?

Raw versus cooked is an interesting debate in the veggie world. You have one camp that says: Go raw, and the other camp that says: Go cooked. I see valid points on both sides. I have become the middle man on this argument for several reasons. I believe in eating at least 50% raw and then the rest steamed or cooked. When you cook certain vegetables, you will get nutrients out of them that you will not get by eating them raw. For instance tomatoes are packed with Lycopene which is great for cancer prevention, however the amount that we get by eating raw is very low in comparison to cooked tomatoes. The same is true with Carrots and other vegetables. The disadvantage of cooking is that we do kill all the enzymes that are attached to the vegetables. This is a study that has barely been looked at by the scientist because of the thousands of different types of enzymes. They do know that enzymes play very critical roles in our daily functions. We are born with a tank full of enzymes. One of their job duties is to help assimilate foods. If we have exhausted all our enzymes from eating all cooked foods, then our digestive system cannot figure out how to process nutrients correctly. That is where the raw really comes into play. If we will eat a portion of raw food at every meal, and preferably before any cooked, then our body can use those enzymes attached to the food to process the cooked food. I no longer take vitamins because I eat a wide range of vegetables, however I will take enzymes on a daily basis to make sure that my body can handle the cooked food portion that I eat. One more negative about cooked food, you can eat too much of it. I find it hard to sit down and eat too many raw vegetables or fruit, but I can pig out on some cooked veggies. If you are trying to lose weight then I would recommend an 85/15 diet. Eating 85% raw and 15% cooked. That will equate to one cooked meal per day and the rest being raw. Again, make sure to eat plenty of raw along with the cooked portion.

Red Cabbage Cole Slaw

- 1 head Red Cabbage
- 1 peeled and cubed cucumber
- 3/4 pine nuts or sunflower seeds
- 2 medium tomatoes
- 1 cubed Avocado
- 1/3 cup olive oil
- 1 minced Jalapeno
- 2 fresh squeezed lemon juice
- 1 tablespoon Dijon mustard
- 1 teaspoon sea salt

In food processor grate or slice red cabbage. Mix together Dijon mustard, olive oil and lemon juice. Pour over salad.

How often can I cheat?

Did you ever ask your teacher this question in school? First, I must say that if you are fighting a disease, especially something like cancer or rheumatoid arthritis I would not cheat period, end of story. That one SAD meal is not worth our life. I have seen people with stage 4 cancer and the doctors had given less than a month to live come back and live a perfect cancer free, pain free life without recurring disease. I have seen people in wheel chairs be able to come out of it and walk miles and miles. I have seen MS patients that were paralyzed in half their body come back and have a career in piano playing on a national level. That makes it worth not having that cheat. We then have to look at the individual. I personally loved cheese. When I transitioned I knew that I could not cheat on cheese or I would fall right back in the SAD diet, so I made that a taboo for me. You know your taboo and stay away from it. If you are a strong person and can limit yourself and jump right back on the horse that you fell off of, then maybe once a month, no more than twice a month. My good friend Dr. Malkmus uses this analogy: Eating animal product is like taking a knife and cutting yourself with it. If you do it continually then you never let your body have a chance to heal. With that said, if you get back on that horse your body should heal in 4 or 5 days and off you go to great health again. It is so hard to give permission to cheat. Every person is different. It is like each person has their own set of weights and balances on their table. Yours might be 4 meals a month before disease can grab hold and take you down or your might be 1 meal a month. I have known people and we all have, that have that "I can eat anything, smoke, drink" and not die until they are hit by a car at 100 years old. That is not the norm folks. I do not recommend that you tempt fate. Especially in today's world that is so much more polluted than before. Learn to enjoy having a body that is superior to any other time in your life. That is how you can maintain and have fun at the same time. Plan on feeling better than you ever have and realize that it is from the way you are now eating and exercising that is making you feel this way.

Spinach Almond Salad

- 6 cups Raw Spinach
- 1/2 cup Parsley - chopped
- 1/4 cup Almond Butter
- 2 tablespoons Flaxseed oil
- 1 tablespoon Apple cider vinegar
- 3 tablespoons Braggs Aminos
- 3 tablespoons Fresh Lemon juice
- 2 cloves Garlic

In blender add almond butter, vinegar, lemon juice, flax oil, braggs and garlic. Blend well. Add a small amount of water if needed. Pour over spinach and serve

Artichoke Salad

- 1 can artichokes
- 1/4 thinly sliced red onion
- 1 cubed Red bell pepper
- 2 heads Broccoli
- 1/4 sliced Black olives
- 1 teaspoon Italian seasoning
- 1 dried Basil
- 1/3 cup Olive Oil
- 2 cloves Garlic
- 1 tablespoon Dijon mustard
- 3 tablespoons Apple cider vinegar

Cut off broccoli stems and use food processor to mince stems. add broccoli tops to food processor and lightly pulse until pieces are about 1/2". Mix Dijon, olive oil, vinegar, garlic and seasonings and pour over salad.

Is it okay to drink coffee and tea?

Wow, you might want to skip over this answer if you are a big caffeine drinker. Caffeine does a lot of ugly things in your body. Yes, you can find the stats out there to find something beneficial from caffeine. Let's look at some of the things that we know caffeine does. Caffeine stimulates your heart and central nervous system. Caffeine dilates your blood veins and makes your blood sludgy by raising fatty acid levels. Coffee and Tea are very acidic contributing to Osteoporosis. Caffeine affects sleeping patterns on most people. I can keep going but I will stop there. If you insist on drinking coffee or tea, I ask you to limit your intake to one cup a day and have it in the AM. If you are wanting a sipping drink that you can drink all day, then I recommend that you take up drinking herbal teas. Now here is something that can be beneficial for you. There are many kinds of herbal teas that have wonderful benefits.

Spinach Lime Salad

- 1/4 cup Grape seed oil or Olive oil
- 2 Limes
- 1/2 teaspoon Sea salt
- 3 cloves Garlic - minced
- 5 cups Raw Spinach

Put spinach in bowl, add oil to spinach and

toss. Add remaining ingredients and toss.

Why do I feel terrible when I transition from animal diet to plant based diet?

This is called detoxing. When you finally take away enough toxins and pollutants from your system, then your body will want to unload and clean house. Your system will have signs of flu or cold or even aches and pains. It depends on where your body stores its toxins. Each person is different. That is why there are different diseases all caused by the same problem, food. Some people will get cancer because that is the weakest area of the body and that is where the body will get the least resistance to store this terrible chemical waste that you have been putting in your body and calling it soda or chips or meat or dairy. You get the picture. If your body is too weak to fight the toxin, it will find a place to store it until the body is strong enough to handle any consequences that it will have by removing it. When we start eating nothing but nutrition, our body jumps at the chance to eliminate these pockets of toxins. That is why we feel sick. This is a great thing. Do not let this deter you from starting. It will typically last for about 2 -3 days and then it is all good after that. You might hit a few detoxes as you go from obese to thin or chemical dependant to freedom of drugs. Each time you will get additional energy and tools after the detox. I can now do much more than I could even 15 years ago. It is amazing to see the body transform into what it was meant to be.

Avocado Salad

- 3 Avocados
- 2 stalks Celery - minced
- 1/2 Sweet Onion - minced
- 1/2 teaspoon Sea salt
- 1/2 teaspoon Tumeric
- 1/2 cup Vegenaise
- 1 Garlic - minced

Cut avocado in half. Take knife and carefully slice to the skin a grid pattern about 1/4". Take a tablespoon and go about 1/2 way deep and remove avocado chunks. You want about 1/4" square chunks. Add remaining ingredients. Blend together without mashing the avocado chinks. Serve on cracker or chip or vegetable slice.

Should I juice?

Juicing is a great way to get maximum nutrients. I am a big advocate of juicing. Juicing allows you to consume nutrients from a pound of each carrots, spinach and celery daily. That is a lot of nutrients! If you are just transitioning to a plant based diet, I recommend that you juice. Most people lack the necessary nutrients when they start a plant based diet. Cravings will also be reduced because juicing satisfies the body by meeting its nutritional needs. They are still thinking in the SAD thought process. Now you have to eat more food. That is what makes this fun. When making your juice, use about 2/3rds carrots and 1/3 greens. You can use any green for the juice. I like celery or spinach or swiss chard. Only make enough for one day unless you have a way to vacuum seal the juice to keep it fresh. Drink 3-8 oz. glasses a day on an empty stomach. You will notice a big energy boost if you do this. If you are diabetic go a 50-50 mixture of greens to carrots and if you can add a teaspoon of flax oil to each serving. This will lower the glycemic index of the drink.

Gazpacho Soup - Cold

- 4 Tomatoes
- 2 Cucumbers - diced
- 2 stalks Celery - minced
- 1/2 Yellow Bell pepper - diced
- 1 Red Bell pepper - diced
- 3 Green onions - minced
- 1 tablespoon Olive oil
- 1 tablespoon Fresh Lime juice
- 1 teaspoon Fresh Lemon juice
- 1 teaspoon Sea salt
- 1 teaspoon Cumin
- 1 teaspoon Chili powder
- 2 cloves Garlic - minced

Place tomatoes in food processor and puree.

Add remaining ingredients and mix. Serve cold

How many times a day should I eat?

The most important thing to remember is that our body needs time to assimilate and eliminate. This should be at least 18 of the 24 hour time period. The amount of times to eat is more determined by our physiques. If you fight weight problems, then you might try 4 or 5 smaller meals with the last meal of the day being all salad. You want to stay away from any starch late at night for several reasons. One is that starch can be converted to fat the easiest. The second reason is that it will keep you awake because of the sugar conversion. If you must eat pasta or baked potato or cooked corn, then do it at lunch time. For dinner, make a great big salad and raw veggie platter and eat until you hurt. The key is low calorie density for dinner.

Sweet Corn Salad

- 6 ears Raw Sweet corn
- 1 Red Bell pepper - diced
- 1 stalk Celery - minced
- 1/4 cup Green olives - sliced
- 1/4 Fresh Cilantro
- 1 tablespoon Olive Oil
- 2 tablespoons Olive Oil

Take a knife and remove corn from cobs. Add remaining ingredients and serve..

Can I drink diet sodas?

Let me try to answer this the best way possible, NO and NO and NO! Diet soda, in my opinion is one of the worst things that you could ever put in your body. They removed the sugar and added the most dangerous poison possible. Did you know that Aspartame is said to have very severe effects on brain tumors, epilepsy, MS, the list goes on and on. This is a known toxin. This is worse than most illegal drugs out there. If people would just read and study what this really does to our body, it should be banned from existence. Aspartame was designed and developed to be an ant poison. Yes to kill ants, that is what it does, kills. Why would we put a known killing agent in our bodies? The other problem with sodas and diet sodas is the Acid content. The average soda is about a 3 on the PH scale we want to be at a 7 on the OH scale. For every point difference, it is to a multiplier of 10 times. So to counteract a cup of soda, you will have to drink 10,000 cups of water. We cannot do this, so our body is very smart. Instead of letting this soda kill us, our body will strip our bones of calcium and counter the acid. Our body is thinking about today, however next year when your bones are brittle and breaking because of lack of calcium in the bones from drinking soda, it might be a good idea to stop drinking the poison.

Lemon Kale Salad

- 4 cups Raw Spinach
- 2 cooked chilled rice or whole wheat Pasta
- 1 large potato - cubed
- 1 Sweet Potato - cubed
- 1/4 Black Olives - sliced
- 1 Red Bell pepper - diced
- 2 stalks Celery - diced
- 1 Yellow Bell pepper - diced

Cook pasta and potatoes and chill. Add celery

and Bell peppers. Blend Thousand Island

dressing or your favorite dressing into

ingredients. Add spinach and black olives.

Lightly stir in spinach and serve.

I am too skinny. What can I do?

First of all, it appears from studies that a skinny person is more apt to be healthy and without disease than a plump person. What you want to concentrate on is building muscle. Start a weight training program. You do not need a gym membership to do this. Start by doing push-ups and sit-ups. If you are weak and cannot do a push-up the correct way, then start by laying flat and come up on your knees rather than your toes. When you can do 15 push-ups this way, then try to graduate to the toes. You need to try and do 4 sets in a row. In other words if you can only do 4 push-ups or sit-ups, than do 4, rest 60 seconds and do another 4, rest another 60 seconds and do it again until you have your 4 sets done. You need to push yourself. After the first set (warm up set) don't stop until you truly cannot do any more. You will begin to see weight gain soon. You can also eat more cooked food than raw food. A person can consume many more calories in cooked food. Sunflower seeds are a good high calorie and high protein food. Make my hummus recipe. Another way to add calories, if you just cannot eat enough volume is to blend your salads. Make up your favorite salad and then put it in a blender and blend it until it is more of a mush or soup. You will find that you can eat about 3 times the amount this way.

Creamy Tomato Soup

- 2 cups water
- 1 cup Pine nuts
- 1/2 teaspoon Cayenne Pepper
- 1 1/2 teaspoons Sea salt
- 1 cup Sun dried tomatoes
- 6 Ripe Tomatoes
- 1/4 cup Fresh Basil or 1 Tbsp dried

Soak Pin nuts and Sun dried tomatoes in water for 30 minutes. Put in blender and mix well. Add remaining ingredients to blender and blend until creamy. Heat using the blender or on stove top.

Can I heat vegetables in a micro wave oven?

No and No. Please get caught up to speed on the dangers of a microwave oven. The Microwave oven will even change the molecular structure of something as simple as water which is H2O. Try this experiment. Go out and buy 2 cheap plants. Water one normally. Take the same amount of water and microwave it. Let it cool and water the other plant. Do this for 2 weeks. You will not need to do it for 2 weeks because the microwave water will kill that plant before 2 weeks are up. Now take a plant that is complicated with molecules and start rearranging molecules. This is not something that we want to put in our bodies. Even worse in animal products. There are many case studies done on microwaves. The best ones are coming out of Europe where they are more health conscious. Let me say it again, NO, do not use a microwave any more for anything. We took ours out and it is now a great place to store fruits and vegetables.

Broccoli Pea Salad

- 2 Large heads Broccoli - minced
- 1 package frozen peas
- 2 stalks Celery - minced
- 1/2 cup Roasted Almonds
- 1 1/2 teaspoons Dill Weed
- 1/2 cup Vegenaise

Remove Broccoli stems and process in food processor until minced. Add broccoli tops and pulse using the S blade until broccoli is about 1/2" pieces. Blend all ingredients. Add 1 Tbsp agave nectar if you want it sweeter.

What is fattening when eating a plant based diet?

Remember oil, no matter if it is olive, coconut or grape seed, is 100% fat. When making dishes or salads, keep this in mind. I find that if I am making somebody else's recipe that I can cut the oil in half, if not eliminate it completely. Oil is the worst. Then comes nuts. Nuts are good for us in a small quantity. A handful of nuts a day are plenty. If you eat a full cup of roasted nuts, you can tip the calorie scale of almost 1000 calories and 56 grams of fat. That is more fat than one day's worth. Pastas, rices and breads; these are foods that are very high in starch and calories. It will put the weight on you rapidly. Cooked corn and white potato are very high in starch. Eat these at lunch time. Fruits are high in sugar, so three to four servings a day should be sufficient. Green vegetables and any vegetables that you are used to seeing in a salad are where you want to eat most of your food from. Try and eat all the different colors as often as possible. This will guarantee that you are getting all the different nutrients that you need.

Spinach Pasta Salad

- 4 cups Raw spinach
- 2 cups cooked, chilled rice or whole wheat pasta
- 1 large potato – cubed
- 1 sweet potato – cubed
- ¼ cup black olives – sliced
- 1 red bell pepper – diced
- 2 stalks celery – diced
- 1 yellow bell pepper – diced

Cook pasta and potatoes and chill. Add celery and bell peppers. Blend thousand island dressing or your favorite dressing into ingredients. Add spinach and black olives. Lightly stir in spinach and serve.

Broccoli Cauliflower Salad

- 1 large head of broccoli – minced
- ½ head of cauliflower – minced
- 1/3 cup fresh lemon juice
- 4 cloves of garlic
- 1 ½ tsp sea salt
- 1 red bell pepper – diced
- ½ cup grape seed oil or olive oil
- 2 carrots – grated or minced
- 1 Tbsp Dijon mustard

Remove stem from Broccoli and place in food processor. Using the S blade, pulse until stems are minced. Remove stems and add broccoli tops. Pulse until pieces are about ½" in size. Put cauliflower in food processor and pulse until minced. Combine all ingredients and serve.

How long until I feel great?

Again every person is different. We run a Lifestyle center outside Branson Mo. Called Hallelujah Acres Lifestyle Center. We see all kinds of people come through our course. The average person will start feeling junky about 24 – 36 hours after eating pure. They will feel sluggish for about 18 hours at our facility. It is shorter than normal because we are pumping them full of incredible nutrients to help give the body the energy to rid itself of the toxins. If you are extremely obese, you will have good days and bad days. The nice thing is you are finally having some good days. Toxins are stored in fat because it is a quick easy way to protect the body from harm. You will find that not only are you losing weight from eating right but now your body will not produce fat cells as protection from what you are putting down the chute.

Rainbow Salad

- ½ head cabbage – diced
- 1 large head of broccoli – minced
- ½ head of cauliflower – minced
- 5 carrots – grated or minced

Mix ingredients together and serve with Sweet Onion salad dressing. For some Fun: Take a wide mug coffee cup and fill the bottom 1/3 with minced cauliflower. Fill the next 1/3 with grated carrots. Finish filling with minced Broccoli. Take a dinner plate and spread about 1/2 cup of minced cabbage on plate. Take coffee mug and turn upside down onto plate. Carefully lift the mug to have a rainbow layered salad. Pour Sweet onion dressing over top and serve.

When can I stop taking my Meds?

You know I cannot legally answer this one. I can tell you testimonies of many people who stopped taking their medications and feel wonderful. I know of one man who got off 17 different medications. I think all of the type 2 diabetics got off their medication after attending a week long course with Hallelujah Acres. Diabetes is an easy one to self monitor since you can check your blood glucose level as you reduce dosages. It takes about 3-4 days to clean up the blood and then it is determined by how over weight you are. The more obese, the longer it might take to see blood sugars or blood pressures reduce. It is always great to hear about people getting off medications that they have been on for decades and now they do not have the horrible side effects that come with drugs.

Carrot Raisin Salad

- 6 carrots – grated or minced
- 1 cup raisins
- 1 cup fresh squeezed orange juice
- 2 tsp cinnamon
- 1 tsp orange zest
- 1 Tbsp Agave Nectar

Combine carrots and raisins in a bowl. In a blender add remaining ingredients and blend well. Pour over salad. You may want to sprinkle some pecans on salad for decoration.

What do I do when we are invited over for dinner?

Your friends will soon learn of your new found love for plant based eating because you will tend to tell everyone how much better you are feeling than they are. Most of our friends try their best to accommodate our lifestyle. The approach I take is I ask them what we will be having and is there anything that I can bring. This gives me a clue to what is on their mind for supper. Many times neighbors and friends do not understand what plant based really is and they tend to add cheese and white flour products. If you ask the question of what are you cooking and what can I bring, you will have a chance to ask if they can leave off the cheese or offer to bring whole grain noodles for them to try. I also bring a big salad. This way if for some reason the meal is mostly animal based, then I have a food source without being obvious that I am not eating their food. Remember "what are we having, can I bring a salad".

Kale Salad

- 2 bunches of kale
- ¼ cup grape seed oil or olive oil
- ¼ cup honey
- 2 cloves garlic
- ½ cup dried cranberries or craisins
- 1 Tbsp pine nuts

Remove kale leaves from stems. Fill food processor no more than half full and pulse until kale is about 1/2" pieces. Place processed kale in bowl and firmly massage with hands for several minutes. Add remaining ingredients and serve.

What can I serve to heavy meat eaters when they come over for dinner?

I used to buy meat and serve them meat to satisfy their desires. I was challenged by a very famous doctor about this and he asked me if I knew someone was a drug addict would I make sure to have drugs available for him. Since then, I do not cater to their whims. Several sure fire recipes that work great for the meat eater is my baked potato with "cheese" and broccoli. I make sure that potato is the biggest I can buy and I pour on the broccoli, green onions, soy based bacon bits and my special "cheese" sauce. The response is incredible. They don't even realize that they just ate without any meat. Another sure fire one is spaghetti. Again, you can doctor it up with veggie burger added to the sauce or sauté some Portobello mushroom chunks and add to the sauce. Remember to use rice or whole wheat noodles.

Broccoli Cabbage Salad

- 2 large heads of broccoli
- ½ head of cabbage
- 4 green onions
- 1 cup of raw sunflower seeds
- ½ cup of slivered almonds
- ½ grape seed oil or olive oil
- ¼ cup honey
- ½ cup fresh lemon juice
- 1 Tbsp Braggs Aminos
- ¼ cup water

Cut stems from broccoli, cut into about 1" pieces & place in food processor with the S blade. Pulse until broccoli is minced. Place broccoli tops in food processor & pulse until about 1/2" pieces. Chunk cabbage & place in food processor & pulse until cabbage is about 1/2" pieces. Slice green onions into small pieces using white and about 1'" of green. Place almonds in oven & broil until golden brown. Add sunflower seeds to ingredients & mix well. Dressing: Add grape seed oil, honey, lemon juice braggs & water & shake or stir well. Pour over salad just prior to serving.

We are big Pizza eaters. What can we do?

I am with you. I love pizza. It is great the first time that you place a phone order for your pizza and you end by saying "oh, and no cheese on the pizza please". You will hear great silence on the other side and then they will make sure that they heard you right and still sound very confused, so help them out on this. Really, it is amazing how good a veggie pizza without cheese can taste. We will go to a pizza place where we can get a whole grain pizza crust and order a veggie lovers pizza without the cheese. Try it, it is great. At home, we will make our own pizzas a couple times a month.

Broccoli and Cauliflower Salad

- 2 large heads broccoli
- 1 head cauliflower – minced
- 1 red bell pepper – diced
- ¼ cup raw sunflower seeds
- ¼ cup raisins
- 1 cup vegenaise
- 3 Tbsp honey
- 2 Tbsp fresh lemon juice
- 1 Tbsp nutritional yeast flakes

Remove stems from broccoli and place in food processor. Using the S blade pulse until stems are minced. Place tops in food processor and pulse until tops are about 1/2" in size. Place cauliflower chunks in food processor and pulse until minced. Mix all ingredients and serve chilled.

How can I tell if the freezer has defrosted and my food is bad?

This is a great little trick that my brother taught me who has a house in Mexico. It is common in some places for power to be off for several hours or even a day. If you have a second home in one of these areas and you return to a freezer with frozen food and do not realize that it is not rotten, you can get deathly sick. The sure way to know is to put a glass with ice cubes in the freezer. Every time you come, be sure to make sure that the ice cubes are still cubes. If you have a glass of ice that is no longer in cube form, then you have had a power failure and you should throw away your food.

Orange Pecan Salad

- 3 heads romaine lettuce
- ½ cup pecans
- 1 small can mandarin oranges
- ½ cup grape seed oil or olive oil
- ¼ cup honey
- 1Tbsp fresh lemon juice
- ½ cup dried cranberries or craisins

Tear romaine lettuce into pieces. Add oranges, pecans and dried cranberries. Mix together oil, lemon juice and honey and pour over salad prior to serving.

Can I eat baked potato chips?

You can eat anything. The question is do you really want to put all those chemicals that come with the baked chip in your body. I just pulled a nutritional fact sheet from a famous brand and the ingredients are: Dried potato, corn starch, sugar, corn oil, salt, soy lecithin and corn sugar. Looking at the ingredients, I don't want to put even one of those in my body, not even dried potato. Many people think they can eat healthy and buy baked. Not true, try something like raw almonds or raw sunflower seeds. My all time favorite is dehydrated Kale chips. This has that incredible cheesy flavor and is all good items.

Cabbage Salad

- 1 head cabbage
- ¼ cup grape seed oil or olive oil
- ¼ cup fresh lemon juice
- 1 tsp sea salt
- 2 Tbsp nutritional yeast flakes

Chunk cabbage and using the S blade, pulse cabbage into small pieces. You can also use the grating blade and grate the cabbage. Mix all ingredients together and serve.

Does attitude affect my health?

When it comes to healing from cancer, most all the oncologists will admit that it will take a positive attitude to survive. This is coming from the doctors that pump chemicals into bodies and they admit that attitude plays a major part. There have been so many studies done with plants that show just by talking to a plant will make it grow better. You can kill a plant by talking rude and cruel to it. Attitude is at the very top of my health scale. We need to learn to be positive in everything we do. We need to learn to encourage people rather than beat them up. When you start praising others, they in turn praise you and this in turn makes you happy which in turn makes people happy around you and in turn: you get where I am going correct? We decide our attitude, no one else. Don't let someone else make that decision for you. It can be the difference between health and disease. Change today. I personally read scripture and find that very life changing. It is a mental decision that you will have to make moment by moment. Try it, you will love it!

Apple Spinach Salad

- 5 cups raw spinach
- 2 apples
- ½ cup honey
- 4 dates
- ¾ cup walnuts
- 3 Tbsp Dijon mustard

Dressing: Pit and soak dates for 20 minutes and drain. In a blender, blend dates, honey, and mustard. Peel and dice apples into about 1/4" chunks. Break walnuts into small pieces. Mix all ingredients and serve.

What about "all in moderation"?

I used to live by this phrase. I used to have aches and pains that I could not explain. I used to take aspirin and sleeping pills. I needed to take blood pressure meds and cholesterol pills and more while living on the "all in moderation" diet. Please do not let yourself go to that diet. It is almost more dangerous than deliberately eating bad. At least when you deliberately do it, you know to stop as soon as you can. The problem about "all in moderation" is that we have been fooled into thinking certain items are okay in "moderation" when in fact it is terrible poison to our bodies. When in doubt, if it flies, swims or walks, don't eat it. Another way to know is if it has a mother, don't eat it. Yes, an egg has a mother.

Spinach Pear Salad

- 6 green onions – minced
- 3 pears
- 2 tsp sea salt
- 1 cup parsley – chopped
- 6 cups raw spinach
- 3 Tbsp Agave Nectar
- ¼ cup grape seed oil or olive oil
- ¼ cup water
- ¼ fresh lemon juice
- ¾ cup pecans

Combine oil, lemon juice, water, agave and salt. blend well. Add pears and let stand for 20 minutes. Add all ingredients, pour dressing over salad and serve.

Can I drink alcohol?

I am not answering this from a spiritual stand point, just my opinion regarding health. Most people have a hard time over indulging on alcohol. Wine can be justified because of polyphenols found in the grape seed along with other nutritional values, however hard liquor is hard to justify. The alcohol content is so high and that kills brain cells and is so hard on the liver and tends to alter our mental state. We want to get to a mental state that is healthy without the use of alcohol. This can be achieved from a pure plant based diet and exercise. A little fact for you: One of the best depression programs out there with a greater than 90% success rate on any type of depression is strictly done with diet, exercise and daily scripture reading, along with no drugs. We need to abide by this same technique for our daily lives and hard alcohol makes it hard to achieve that goal. Did I answer your question? Sometimes I have to skirt the obvious answer.

Sweet Potato Salad

- 4 cups sweet potato
- 1 small fresh pineapple
- ½ cup pecans
- ½ cup dried cranberries or craisins
- ½ cup vegenaise
- 2 Tbsp Agave Nectar
- 2 Tbsp fresh lemon juice
- 1 tsp lemon zest

Peel sweet potatoes. Using the grating blade in your food processor, process sweet potatoes. Dice pineapple into about 1/4" chunks. Mix all ingredients together and serve.

Sweet Broccoli Salad

- 3 heads of broccoli
- 1 cup raw sunflower seeds
- ½ sweet onion – sliced
- ½ cup raisins
- ½ red bell pepper – minced
- 2 Tbsp apple cider vinegar
- ¼ tsp sea salt
- ¼ cup water
- 1 cup cashews
- ¼ cup Agave Nectar

Dressing: Add cashews, salt, vinegar, water and agave and blend well. Remove stems from Broccoli and place in food processor with the S blade. Pulse until minced. Place broccoli tops in food processor and pulse until about 1/2" pieces. Combine all ingredients and serve.

Zucchini Salad

- ½ cup vegenaise
- 2 Tbsp apple cider vinegar
- 1 tsp sea salt
- 4 green onions
- 1 red bell pepper – diced
- 1 Tbsp Dijon mustard
- 1 Tbsp Agave Nectar
- 3 zucchinis
- 2 stalks of celery – diced
- 2 carrots

Chop green onions, dice bell pepper, peel and cube zucchini in about 1/4" cubes. Mince celery. Peel carrots. Place in blender and cover with water. Pulse blender until carrots are minced. Drain carrots. Place all ingredients together, mix well and serve.

Apple Spinach Salad

- 2 carrots – diced
- 2 stalks of celery – diced
- 2 apples
- ½ head of cauliflower – minced
- 1 head broccoli – minced
- ¼ cup raisins
- ½ cup cashews
- 2 cups raw spinach
- ½ cup grape seed oil or olive oil
- ¼ cup apple cider vinegar
- ¼ cup Agave Nectar
- 1 tsp sea salt
- 1 clove garlic – minced
- 2 Tbsp fresh lemon juice
- ½ cup water

Blend oil, water, vinegar, agave, salt, garlic and lemon. Mince broccoli and cauliflower in food processor, Mince carrots and celery in food processor. Dice apples. Combine ingredients and add dressing. Place a bed of spinach on plate and put mixture on spinach and serve.

Heart of Palm Salad

- 2 cucumbers – diced
- ¼ red onion – diced
- 1 red bell pepper
- 1 can Heart of Palm
- 1 can quartered artichoke
- 4 medium ripe tomatoes
- 1 can black olives – sliced
- ½ tsp dried oregano
- 2 Tbsp fresh lemon juice
- 2 Tbsp olive oil
- 1 head romaine lettuce

Broccoli Bac-un Salad

- 2 heads of broccoli
- 3 green olives – sliced
- 1 cup grapes
- ½ cup slivered almonds
- ½ cup vegenaise
- 2 Tbsp soy bac-un bits
- 1 tsp sea salt

Remove stems from broccoli and place in food processor. Using the S blade, pulse the broccoli until it is minced. Place broccoli tops in processor and pulse until pieces are 1/2" in size. Slice grapes into 4ths. Toast almonds in oven. Mix all ingredients and serve chilled.

Sweet and Sour Kale

- ½ cup Agave Nectar
- ½ cup fresh lemon juice
- ¼ cup grape see oil or olive oil
- 1 tsp sea salt
- 1tsp celery salt
- 4 bunches of kale
- 2 stalks of celery – diced
- ½ red bell pepper – diced
- 3 carrots – grated or minced
- 2 apples or mangos

Dressing: Blend together agave, lemon juice, olive oil, salt and celery seed. Remove kale leaves from stems. Fill food processor half full with kale. Using the S blade pulse until pieces are 1/2" in size. Place kale in bowl and firmly massage with your hands for 2 minutes. Dice apples or mangos, celery, bell pepper and carrots. Mix together and serve.

House Salad

- 3 heads romaine lettuce
- 1 red bell pepper – sliced thin
- 2 ripe tomatoes
- 1 avocado
- 5 green onions – minced
- 10 black olives
- 1 carrot – diced
- 1 yellow bell pepper – sliced thin

Tear romaine lettuce into small pieces, dice tomatoes into 1/2" cubes, cube avocado into 1/2" cubes by carefully slicing the avocado in the half shell and remove meat with a spoon. Slice olives. Slice red bell and yellow bell pepper in thin slices. Mix all in a salad bowl and add your favorite dressing.

Beet Salad

- 2 cups diced carrots
- 2 cups diced beets
- 2 heads romaine lettuce
- 1 cup chopped cabbage
- 1 red bell pepper – diced
- ¼ cup chopped parsley
- ¼ cup olive oil
- 2 Tbsp red wine vinegar
- 1 tsp sea salt
- ¼ cup diced onion
- ¼ cup vegenaise
- 1/8 tsp ground pepper
- ¼ cup sliced green olives (optional)

Bring some water to a boil and add carrots and cook for 5 minutes. Drain and cool. Mix all ingredients together and serve.

Red Leaf and Beet Salad

- 1 large head red leaf lettuce
- 1 large beet
- ¼ cup sliced green olives
- ¼ cup sliced Italian peppers
- ½ cup vegenaise
- ¼ cup nutritional yeast flakes
- 3 Tbsp red wine vinegar

Wash and cut red leaf into bit size pieces. Peel and Slice or shred beet. Slice peppers thinly. Slice avocado and olives. Mix Vegenaise, Nutritional Yeast and vinegar. Dress salad and serve.

Taco Salad

- ½ head white cabbage
- ½ head of broccoli
- ½ head of cauliflower
- 2 celery sticks
- 4 green onions
- ¼ red onion sliced thin
- ½ cup sliced black olives
- ½ tsp onion powder
- 1 can diced or stewed tomatoes
- 2 pickled jalapeños
- 2 sliced avocados
- ½ tsp garlic powder
- ½ tsp sea salt
- 2 Tbsp Braggs Aminos
- 2 Tbsp apple cider vinegar
- 2 Tbsp olive oil
- 3 Tbsp fresh cilantro
- 1 lime

Slice avocados, black olives and set aside. Using a food processor dice all remaining ingredients. Add can of diced tomato. Add all remaining ingredients. Toss and serve. Squeeze lime over salad before serving.

MAIN DISHES

I want to lose weight quickly. How can I do it?

Well, it is not best to lose weight quickly, however sometimes there are events that we want to look good for and really want to lose some lbs. The best way is to eat 100% raw and double your water intake and double your exercise routine. This will peel the weight off you. If you find that you are detoxifying too fast (because this is also a detoxify remedy), try doing 2 coffee enemas a day for 3 days in a row. You can learn all about enemas on the web.

I love Cheese. What can I do?

I was a huge cheese lover. That is also why I was 55lbs overweight and had blood pressure of 210 over 110. Cheese is very hard to duplicate. I have several recipes and you can find many on the web, however they really do not replace cheese. This is one area where you really need to bite the bullet and stop. You cannot cheat on cheese and have "just a little slice". Not only is it then impossible to lose the addiction, but it is pounding terrible toxins into your body and they stay there for some time. With that said, I do have a great cheese sauce to put over baked potatoes or Broccoli or pasta. It is so simple and great tasting. Take 1 cup of vegenaise (vegan mayonnaise) and ½ cup Nutritional Yeast flakes and about 1/3 cup water. Blend and enjoy. It is great.

Beef Stroganoff

- 1 package portabella mushrooms – sliced
- 4 Tbsp fresh lemon juice
- 3 large cloves of garlic
- 1 sweet onion – diced
- 2 Tbsp tamari
- 2 tsp sea salt
- 4 Tbsp coconut oil
- 1 ½ cups vegenaise
- 3 Tbsp nutritional yeast

Sauté diced onions, minced garlic and sliced mushrooms in coconut oil for about 4 minutes or until onions become transparent. Add remaining ingredients and simmer for 3 minutes. Serve over rice noodles. For Diabetes - increase the mushrooms and reduce the pasta. weight - only use 1/4 cup vegenaise and add 3/4 cup water and 2 tsp.

It hurts to exercise. Do I have to?

Yes, the answer is yes. A wonderful tool to buy is a rebounder. I have a sheet of paper that has 50 reasons to rebound. The biggest reason in my book is that while you exercise you also are dumping your lymph nodes. Our lymph nodes do not have a pump so we need to bounce to drain them. When we were youngsters, we were bouncing all the time. Now that we are older we do not bounce, so this is very important to do. Start slow and make yourself increase every day. I had one lady on a walker that started bouncing for only 30 seconds at a time and in a week was up to 5 minutes. Guess what? She was not using a walker after 2 weeks. If you cannot walk at all, then use your arms and start exercising with them. Start by doing circles and continue until you can use weights. We need to exercise. We need to make that blood pump through our veins. We were not designed to go in slow motion all the time. When we move blood faster and pump it harder, it strengthens the heart muscle and at the same time starts cleaning the veins. Please do not talk yourself out of this. Even if you think a little won't help, it will. Just keep pushing yourself to add a few more seconds of bouncing or walk a few more steps or lift a heavier weight. It will pay big dividends.

Potato and Corn Chowder

- 1 medium onion – diced
- 1 clove garlic
- ¼ tsp cumin
- 3 cups water or vegetable broth
- ¼ tsp nutmeg
- 4 cups fresh or frozen corn
- 2 potatoes – diced into ½" cubes
- 1 sweet potato – diced into ¼" cubes
- ¼ cup nutritional yeast
- 1 cup coconut milk
- 1 tsp sea salt

Sauté onion and garlic in coconut oil for about 3 minutes. Add remaining ingredients and simmer for 30 minutes.

What about Omega 3 fish oil?

Omega-3 fatty acid supplements are made from either fish oils or from plant oils such as flax seed oil, but there are some structural differences between the two sources. Fish oil contains two long-chain fatty acids called docosahexaenoic acid (DHA) and eicosapentaenoic acid (EPA), which are the forms of omega-3s that your body uses for a variety of purposes. Flax and other plant oils contain alpha-linolenic acid (ALA), which is also an omega-3 fatty acid, but is slightly different from EPA and DHA. Your body should be able to convert the ALA to DHA or EPA. Algal oil, which is made from ocean algae, is the one plant source of omega-3 fatty acids that contains pre-formed DHA. Algal oil is also sold as a dietary supplement.

Broccoli Potato Soup

- 4 cups water
- 2 heads broccoli
- 3 stalks celery
- 1 Tbsp garlic powder
- ½ cup nutritional yeast
- 5 large potatoes – diced into ½" cubes
- 3 carrots – diced
- 1 Tbsp onion powder
- ½ tsp sea salt
- ½ tsp cayenne pepper

Combine all ingredients in a large pot and simmer for 45 minutes.

Secrets to Great Eating

Eating healthy is a simple, easy to understand process…but still, there are lots of questions about myths and "old wives tales" out there regarding how to eat right. In this section we've provided lots of helpful answers and secrets to better eating. Hopefully, after you read this section, you'll better understand the truth about great eating. Enjoy!

What items should I buy organic?

If you are on a budget, the first items to buy organic will be your root vegetables. This is where the most toxins can enter into the vegetable. I buy organic carrots, onions and potatoes. The next items would be fruit. Most fruit is sprayed with heavy chemicals. If you can't buy organic, then peel the fruit before eating.

Veggie Burgers

- 1 pint baby Portobello mushrooms
- 2 Tbsp olive oil
- 1 tsp olive oil
- 1 tsp coriander
- 1 tsp balsamic vinegar
- ¾ cups walnuts
- 1 medium onion
- ½ red bell pepper
- 2 cups uncooked oatmeal
- 2 stalks celery
- 3 cloves garlic
- 1 Tbsp Dijon mustard
- 1 ½ cups wheat germ (add more if too wet)
- 1 cup warm water (add more if too dry)
- 1 tsp sea salt
- 1 tsp oregano
- 3 Tbsp nutritional yeast
- 2 Tbsp bakon hickory flavoring (optional)

Combine spices & liquid. Add processed veggies & let stand for 5 min. Mix all dry ingredients well. Combine all ingredients & form patties. Brown in skillet in grape seed oil.

How to dice an onion:

Cut both ends off your onion. Remove the outer peeling of the onion. Stand the onion on end and slice the onion in half. Now lay the onion on the flat side and make slices going with the grain of the onion. Slice every ¼" so you have many long slices of onion. Now hold the onion together with your hand and rotate the onion 90 degrees. Now slice the onion going the other direction, against the grain. This will give you nice little ¼" squares of onion. To mince, just make closer cuts. You can use this same process with tomatoes.

Navy Bean Soup

- 2 cups dry navy beans
- 6 cups water
- 1 Tbsp olive oil
- 2 cloves minced garlic
- 2 tsp sea salt
- ½ tsp cumin
- 2 Tbsp nutritional yeast
- 2 cups chopped kale
- 1 medium onion – diced
- 1 large potato – diced into ½" cubes
- 1 sweet potato – diced into ¼" cubes

Cook beans until tender. A pressure cooker is a very fast and good way to cook beans. Sauté garlic and onions in olive oil for about 3 minutes. Add all ingredients to cooked beans and simmer for an additional 30 minutes.

Stuffed Bell Peppers

- 1 ½ cups uncooked brown rice
- 3 cups water
- 1 medium onion – diced
- 1/3 cup nutritional yeast
- 2 tsp sea salt
- ½ cup wild rice
- ½ cup grated carrots
- ½ tsp dill weed
- 2 red bell peppers – sliced in half
- 3 Tbsp coconut oil
- 1 cup vegenaise
- ½ cup water

Cook brown rice and wild rice separately. Sauté onions, garlic and carrots in coconut oil for about 4 minutes. Remove seeds from bell pepper halves. Mix vegenaise, nutritional yeast, dill weed and 1/2 cup water. Pour about 3/4 of mixture and mix in with both rice's. Place bell peppers in baking dish. Mound rice mixture into bell pepper halves. Pour remaining vegenaise mixture over top. Place in oven for 30 minutes at 350 degrees.

I am really craving meat. What can I do?

Try making my Beaf Strogonaff recipe with Portabella muchrooms and pasta noodles. Another great deterrent is to take zuchinni and bread in onion powder and fry in a small amount of grape seed or coconut oil. Use some salt and pepper to taste. You can do this with mushrooms also. Try my pot roast recipe.

Portobella Pot Roast

- 4 portobella mushrooms
- 8 potatoes – cut into 1" cubes
- 6 carrots
- 3 Tbsp onion powder
- 1 tsp sea salt
- 2 Tbsp coconut oil
- 3 sweet onions
- 2 tsp garlic powder
- ½ tsp black pepper
- ½ tsp Braggs or Tamari sauce
- 2 cups water

Mix onion powder, garlic powder, pepper and salt on a plate. Coat mushroom with mixture. Sprinkle Braggs or Tamari on bottom side of mushrooms. Brown mushrooms in coconut oil in skillet. Slice onion into 1/4" thick rings. Slice carrots into quarters. Cube mushrooms into 1" cubes. Add all ingredients into baking dish. Add water. Sprinkle remaining onion powder mixture over vegetables. Cover and place in oven for 90 minutes at 375 degrees.

What can I eat for lunch if I am away from home?

My choices are 5 times greater than a S.A.D. eater. By the way, S.A.D. stands for standard American diet. Myself, I like to go to a Health Food store. Most all your larger Health food stores now have wonderful salad bars, hot food bars, soups, etc. You do need to be a little cautious because some serve dairy products in their food such as cheese, butter or sour cream. Please stay away from these. If you don't have a health food store, then I would go to a grocery store and buy an avocado, red bell pepper and a piece of sweet corn. Learn to always pack a knife, fork and spoon, and sea salt. When you first start on this journey, you might feel that you still need a piece of bread to consider it a meal. Buy some healthy crackers. Just don't eat the whole box at your first lunch. Or buy some Pita bread and stuff that avocado and bell pepper in it and you will think you died and went to heaven. There is always the backup of a sub shop. If you do this, order a veggie sandwich on whole grain bread and no mayo. Mustard is a good dressing along with some vinegar and oil. Most of the preprocessed salads at your fast food establishments have tons of mayo or cheese or MSG, etc. I try to stay away from any exotic salads. If you order a fast food salad, then get the basic salad and a side of Balsamic dressing. Oh, throw away the croutons, don't temp yourself. They have tons of toxins built in them.

Coconut Curry Vegetables

- 3 heads broccoli
- 2 red bell peppers – cubed
- 4 cups cooked brown rice
- 1 sweet onion – cubed
- 1 package sliced mushrooms
- 2 tsp coconut milk
- 2 tsp curry powder
- 2 Tbsp Braggs or Tamari Sauce
- 2 Tbsp Raw Agave Nectar
- 2 Tbsp arrow root or corn starch
- ¼ cup water
- 3 carrots – thinly sliced

Sauté onion and mushroom in olive oil. Steam broccoli, bell peppers and carrots for 10 minutes. Combine coconut milk, Braggs, nectar, curry powder and place in sauce pan on stove. Heat to almost boiling. Add arrow to water and stir. Add arrow root liquid to sauce pan and heat until it become thick. Pour mixture over vegetables and serve.

Spaghetti Blush

- 4 cloves garlic
- 1 medium onion – diced
- 2 tsp oregano
- 2 veggie burgers – frozen (optional)
- 2 tsp basil
- 2 Tbsp olive oil
- 2 20 oz cans of tomatoes in tomato juice
- 2 bay leaves
- ¾ cup vegenaise

Sauté onions and garlic for about 3 minutes. Remove and put in sauce pan. Blend tomatoes in blender and add to sauce pan. Simmer for 30 minutes until sauce is reduced and thicker. Crumble or dice veggie burgers. Brown veggie burgers and add to sauce. Add vegenaise. Cook rice or whole wheat noodles to al dente. Rinse noodles. Place noodles on plate. Cover with blush sauce.

I get tired in the afternoon. How can I get energy?

The best way to overcome the 3:00 sleepy time is to go for a 10 – 15 minute power walk at 2:45. Eat a banana and some pineapple and get your blood pumping. I also will make a smoothie or take a good green drink. If you are at work, sneak into the bathroom or a room and do 30 jumping jacks. You will be amazed at how exercise will wake you up.

Tuscan Pasta

- 1 red bell pepper – sliced
- 1 sweet onion – sliced
- ½ cup olive oil
- 1/3 cup green olives or capers
- 2 tsp dried basil
- 1 yellow bell pepper
- 1 package sliced mushrooms
- 5 cloves garlic – minced
- 3 roma tomatoes
- 1 Tbsp balsamic vinegar

Slice all vegetables in thin ¼ slices. Sauté all ingredients except tomatoes in 1/4 cup water and 2 Tbsp olive oil for 10 minutes. With 1 minute left, add tomatoes and remaining olive oil. Serve over pasta.

Zucchini Parmesans

Get out your frozen veggie burgers for this one.

- 4 medium zucchinis
- 2 28 oz cans of roma tomatoes
- 4 cloves garlic
- 4 Tbsp olive oil
- 2 veggie burgers – frozen (optional)
- 1 Tbsp basil
- 2 Tbsp nutritional yeast
- ¾ cup vegenaise
- 3 Tbsp onion powder
- 1 tsp sea salt

Sauté garlic in olive oil for about 3 minutes. Add tomatoes and Basil and simmer for 30 minutes to reduce liquid. Remove half the sauce to another pan. Add 2 veggie burgers chopped up into small pieces. Add vegenaise and Nutritional yeast. Peel zucchini and slice into about 3/8" thick slices. Coat the zucchini in onion powder and sea salt. Brown the zucchini in olive oil for about 3 minutes per side or until brown. Place browned zucchini on plate and cover with sauce.

I am allergic to certain vegetables. What can I do?

Food allergies are actually caused from the animal fat in our blood with the exception of sulfur allergies. I would suggest that you stay away from the vegetable that you are currently allergic to and eat a total plant based diet for one week. After the week you will be able to bring those foods into your diet and the allergies will be gone. If for some reason you have some allergic reaction, then reduce the initial amount and work up to a full serving after about 2 weeks.

Fajitas

- 3 cloves garlic – minced
- 1 package sliced portobella mushrooms
- 1 poblano chile or 1 can green chiles
- ½ tsp sea salt
- ¾ tsp dried or 2 Tbsp fresh cilantro
- 1 medium lime
- ½ tsp cayenne
- 2 roma tomatoes
- 1 onion – sliced
- 1 red bell pepper – sliced
- 1 broccoli head
- ¼ tsp cumin
- 2 tsp hickory flavoring (optional)
- ½ cup olive oil
- 3 jalapeños (optional)
- ¼ head cabbage

Sauté all ingredients except tomatoes in olive oil for about 10 minutes. Add tomatoes and simmer for 1 minute. Serve with warm corn tortillas and refried beans. Dice 2 roma tomatoes, 1 sweet onion, 3 fresh jalapeños (optional), ¼ head of cabbage for garnish.

I hate the taste of most vegetables. What can I do?

Our taste buds are formed in about 21 days. If you will just hang in there for 3 weeks, all your taste buds will adapt to your new lifestyle. All the fat that has coated your tongue and changed your taste buds will sluff off and you will be able to enjoy the real taste of vegetables. Another way is to initially use dressings with strong flavors. For instance my sweet onion salad dressing recipe will mask many flavors. You can use my cheesy sauce recipe for cooked vegetables. Find a sauce and dressing that you like and keep it handy until your taste buds change.

Chili

- 2 cups dried kidney beans
- 1 cup dried pinto beans
- 9 cups water
- 1 28 oz can diced tomatoes
- ½ tsp cayenne pepper
- 1 tsp cumin
- 4 cloves garlic – minced
- ¼ tsp dried sage
- 2 Tbsp chili powder

In a pressure cooker add the beans and water. Once the pressure cooker gets up to pressure, reduce heat to low for 45 minutes. You can also slow cook your beans the conventional way. Just make sure to give yourself enough time to cook the beans. Sauté' the garlic and onions in olive oil for 3 minute or until the onions are transparent. Add tomatoes, beans and all seasonings and simmer for 15 minutes.

How much water should I drink?

Rule of thumb is half your body weight in ounces. If you weight 150lbs, then you should be drinking 75 ounces of water a day. That is 2 quarts and 1 cup of water per day. It is a good habit to drink a few glasses of water as soon as you awake in the morning. This gets your body hydrated first thing in the morning helping set your organs to function better.

What can I drink when eating?

The best answer is nothing. You want to refrain from drinking if possible for at least 20 minutes prior to eating and then for at least one hour after eating. Drinking fluids has a tendency to dilute the stomach acids that help break down the foods that we eat.

Veggie Wrap

- ¼ cup grape seed oil or olive oil
- ¼ cup Braggs Aminos
- 1 tsp cumin
- 2 tsp coriander
- 2 Tbsp balsamic vinegar
- 2 portobella mushrooms – diced
- 1 red bell pepper – thinly sliced
- 1 cup broccoli – minced
- 2 cloves garlic
- 1 cup pine nuts or cashews
- ½ cup raw sunflower seeds
- 3 Tbsp apple cider vinegar
- ¼ onion – minced
- ½ sweet onion – sliced

Make a marinate sauce with the oil, Braggs, cumin, coriander, garlic and balsamic vinegar. Add diced mushrooms, onions and bell pepper to marinate and let stand for at least 10 minutes. Make a nut paste using the pine nuts, sunflower seeds, apple cider vinegar, and onion. Place all ingredients in a blender and blend well. Add a small amount of water if needed. Take a tortilla or large leaf lettuce of your choice and lay flat. Spread a layer of nut paste on wrap. Add vegetables from marinate. Add broccoli. Roll edges up on wrap and serve.

I love milk. What can I do?

I have to get on my milk wagon for a moment. DON'T Drink Milk!!! There are now so many studies that milk is terrible for you. Your chances of breaking a bone is 3.7 times greater if you are a milk drinker. Your chance of Osteoporosis increases many fold from drinking milk. Be sure and let any new mothers know to not let their kids drink milk prior to age 2. It has been proven that Type 1 diabetes is caused by amino acids in cow's milk. If they have to supplement and insist on some kind of animal, then go with goat, however almond or rice milk also work. You can make your own almond milk very easy. Buy raw almonds. Add 1 cup of almonds to 1 quart of water and blend on high for 1 minute. Take a cheese cloth and strain the milk, or if you like pulp, just drink it that way. You can then make some great cheese recipes or spreads with the pulp from the milk. Stay away from Soy milk. You will acclimate to this quickly. Just like going from whole milk to 2% way back when. Search YouTube for Almond Milk to learn tricks.

Bruschetta

- 5 medium ripe tomatoes
- ½ sweet onion – minced
- ½ cup fresh basil or 1 Tbsp dried basil
- 1 tsp sea salt
- ½ yellow bell pepper – diced
- ½ cup olive oil
- 2 Tbsp Braggs Aminos
- 1 tsp apple cider vinegar
- ½ tsp cumin
- ½ tsp coriander
- 6 pieces whole grain bread
- 4 cloves garlic – minced

Dice tomatoes into small pieces. Mince onion. Add all ingredients and let stand for 20 minutes. Toast Whole grain bread. Mound mixture on toast and slice in half diagonally. Serve.

How can I know if I am getting enough protein?

Edema and ridges on finger and toe nails are signs of protein deficiency. To my knowledge, there are no domestic deaths due to protein deficiency. That includes all vegans and vegetarians. We have been bamboozled to think that we need all this protein to maintain, when in fact excessive protein is causing the greater majority of all diseases. The China Study documents a 30 year study in China with many villages that never ate meat or dairy and guess what? They had no cancer, heart disease, osteoporosis, diabetes, on and on. They did not die of protein deficiency. If you will eat a well rounded amount of vegetables, nuts and seeds along with legumes, you will get plenty of protein. If you have a youth wanting to build muscle and is still growing, then you can add additional seed like sunflower seeds and raw soy beans and more legumes. Greens are a very dense source of healthy protein.

Cheesy Baked Potato

- 4 large baking potatoes
- ¾ cup vegenaise
- 1/3 cup nutritional yeast flakes
- ¼ cup water

Coat potatoes with olive oil and sprinkle with salt. Place in oven at 400 degrees for 1 hour. Remove potatoes and slice down the center and push on the sides to open the potato. Mix vegenaise, yeast and water and shake well. Pour mixture over potatoes. You can add steamed broccoli and minced green onions and soy Bac-un bits to make a Loaded potato.

Should I continue to take my vitamins?

I used to have a vitamin store and I had a machine that could test to see if the vitamin that a person was taking actually was absorbing into their body. The sad truth is that less than 10% really did absorb. Then you have the problem of balancing vitamins or minerals. I stopped consuming vitamins in 2008 and I feel so much better than before. Trying to balance your body using vitamins is like trying to build a jet liner from a convenience store. For example there are more than 1200 known enzymes in broccoli alone. They have only categorized about 200 of them so far. How can we think that by taking 12 – 20 different vitamins or minerals that we are going to balance such a sophisticated body. We more than not actually get our body out of balance by taking vitamins. Most of the nutrients put into the vitamins cannot be absorbed by our body and a few can so now we are getting off balance thus making our body fight this new problem of imbalance.

Baked Cabbage Rolls

- 1 head cabbage
- 4 carrots
- 2 heads broccoli
- ½ head cauliflower
- ½ sweet onion
- 1 red bell pepper
- 1 cup vegenaise
- 1/3 cup nutritional yeast flakes
- ¼ cup water
- 3 cloves garlic
- 3 Tbsp olive oil
- 2 tsp sea salt

Remove 8 large cabbage leaves and place in large pan with 1 cup of water and steam for 10 minutes. Set aside. In your food processor using the S blade mince all vegetables. Do vegetable individually to obtain proper consistency. Take about 2 cups of cabbage and mince in food processor. In large pan sauté all vegetables in olive oil for 10 minutes or until tender. Mix vegenaise, yeast flakes, salt and water and shake well. Pour 3/4 cup into vegetable mixture. Lay your large cabbage leaf flat and put about 1/2 cup of mixture onto leaf. Roll leaf and place in baking dish. Pour remaining sauce over cabbage rolls. Bake at 350 for 15 minutes.

What supplements should I take?

The beauty of a plant based diet is that if you eat a well rounded variety of plants with different colors, then you are getting the best source of vitamins that you could ask for. This is exactly how God intended us to get vitamins. The scientists are smart but they are light years away from understanding the mechanics of enzymes and how they interact with vitamins and minerals and micronutrients and on and on. Studies have shown that most Americans are deficient in 2 nutrients. The first was in sunshine or vitamin D. Our body needs vitamin D to synthesize most vitamins and minerals. Vitamin D plays a major role with daily functions such as mood swings, depression, nervous system and clarity of mind. The best type is an oil base D3 vitamin. The other nutrient is B12 with folic acid. Because we have become germaphobics, we now have become B12 deficient. B12 is found from the dirt on vegetables or other items. We now wash and disinfect everything we touch and have lost that form of contact. You will want to buy a sublingual version because it is hard to absorb this vitamin. Place the pill under your tongue and let it absorb through your mouth using your saliva.

Coconut Vegetables

- 1 yellow bell pepper – thinly sliced
- 1 zucchini – diced
- 1 yellow squash – diced
- ½ sweet onion – thinly sliced
- ½ cup raisins
- 2 cloves garlic – minced
- ½ cup coconut flakes – optional
- 3 Tbsp Agave Nectar
- ½ cup celery – diced
- ¼ pine nuts
- ½ tsp sea salt
- 2 uncooked brown rice
- 1 28 oz diced tomatoes
- ½ cup diced pineapple

Cook Brown rice. Dice all ingredients and put in a sauce pan. Add tomatoes with juice. Put coconut flakes in blender and blend to very small pieces. Add coconut, salt and agave. Add enough water to cover vegetables. Bring to boil. Simmer until the liquid is reduced, about 30 minutes. Serve over brown rice.

Can dogs and cats eat a plant based diet?

Yes, I have several friends that have put their pets on a plant based diet. Our dog is about 60/40. He loves veggies but I still buy regular dog food to supplement his diet. I do not have the time to prepare him a proper diet. It should have cooked brown rice and lentils along with other vegetables. If you look at the true nature of the dog, I do not think that it was designed to be a vegan. Not only does it have large canine teeth but the stomach is different than ours and the acids are stronger than ours. Same with cats, they have a much shorter stomach and it is smooth inside without the little ripples like ours have. Another observation to think about is this. Put an infant and a dog in a room with a rabbit. Observe which one starts salivating and chasing the rabbit. Put a cat and a girl in a room with a mouse and watch what happens. That is born into animals that are not plant based eaters. I personally don't think we should try to change them.

Stir Fry Noodles

- 2 heads broccoli
- ½ pound spinach
- ½ tsp onion powder
- ½ tsp garlic powder
- 1 pacakge Whole wheat or rice spaghetti noodles
- 1 tsp sea salt
- 3 Tbsp nutritional yeast flakes

Add 2 Tbsp olive oil to a frying pan. Slice broccoli stems thinly and add to hot oil. Add 1/2 tsp. Garlic powder and 1/2 tsp onion powder. Sauté until stems start to darken. Sauté broccoli tops and spinach until tender. Set aside. Boil noodles, drain and set aside. Add remaining oil, garlic and onion powder to fry pan. Heat pan and add noodles to hot oil. Stir fry for several minutes. Mix vegetables with noodles and serve.

Jim Bakker's Bean Burger

- 6 cups cooked lentils
- 2 cups crushed walnuts
- ½ cup nutritional yeast
- 2 tsp sea salt
- 3 Tbsp olive oil
- 2 Tbsp crushed red pepper
- 1 Tbsp cumin
- 2 Tbsp mustard
- 1 cup grated carrots
- 1 onion diced
- 12 cloves garlic minced
- 2 cups raw oats
- 1 cup soy or rice milk
- 2 Tbsp cilantro

Process all ingredients in a food processor until minced.

BREADS & ROLLS

What kind of bread can I eat?

The only bread that should ever go in your mouth is whole grain bread. Do not be deceived by Whole Wheat bread. Make sure that is whole grain. With whole grain you will not get the "enriched with vitamins" label. You do not want that. Anything besides whole grain is a big toxin to your body. There is no fiber and no nutrition and then it just plugs up your whole system from functioning the way it is supposed to. If you go to a sub shop for a plant based only sandwich, be sure and get whole grain bread. If they don't have it, then get a salad instead. If you get a salad, be sure to tell them no croutons! They are made from white bread and butter and typically MSG.

Whole Grain Bread

- 3 ¼ cups warm water
- 2/3 cup fine ground lentils
- 1/3 cup coarse ground oatmeal
- 2/3 cup ground barley
- 2/3 cup ground flax seed
- 3 Tbsp yeast
- 3 Tbsp molasses
- 2 Tbsp honey
- ½ cup whole wheat flour

Warm the mixing bowl and fill with luke warm water. Add molasses and honey and mix well. Add 1/4 cup whole wheat flour and yeast. Mix well, and let stand for 5 minutes or until you see bubbles forming. Add ground lentils, ground Barley and ground flax. Let stand for 5 minutes. Add additional whole wheat flour until dough is barley sticky. Separate in half and make 2 dough balls. Pour oat flour on counter and knead into dough. Form dough into 2 loaves and place into non stick bread pans. Let rise until dough doubles on size. Carefully place bread in oven at 400 degrees for 10 minutes. Reduce heat to 350 and bake an additional 20 minutes.

DESSERTS

Smoothie a Day!

As a special treat every day you can get a nice cool smoothie and still create health and wellness. Below is a recipe you can use to get energy, fresh starts and a healthy dose of vitamins and natural sugars. You can shake and eat between breakfast and lunch for a pick me up.

I have a sweet tooth. How do I satisfy it?

Another touchy area here. If a person has a craving for illegal drugs, what should we do? Do we allow them to have it because their body is calling for it? Sugar addiction is sugar addiction. We should not be addicted to anything, including sugar. If you don't think it is an addiction, just stop all sugars and watch what happens. We need to reset our taste buds. This can be no fun to do, but might be the number one best thing that you will ever do for your body. Once you have reset your taste buds, your sugar cravings will be gone and you will enjoy the sweetness of fruits and vegetables much more. By eliminating the sugars from your body this will help your entire immune system. For every teaspoon of sugar you ingest, it shuts down your immune system for several hours leaving you susceptible to viruses, germs, bacterias, on and on. It also causes inflammation. If you want to get rid of that lower back pain try stopping caffeine and sugar for 2 weeks and watch the pain go away.

Apple Pie

- 2 cups almonds
- ½ cup dates
- 2 Tbsp ground flax seed
- 4 apples
- 1 tsp cinnamon
- 2 tsp fresh lemon juice
- ¼ tsp sea salt
- ¼ cup honey
- 4 dates
- ½ cup raisins

To make the crust: Soak 1/2 cup pitted dates for 20 minutes in water. Drain dates. Put 2 cups almonds in food processor and process until minced. Add drained dates and 2 tablespoons of ground flax seed. Mix in food processor until mixture is blended and minced. Press mixture in pie dish. Filling: Soak 4 pitted dates in water for 20 minutes and drain. Peel apples and remove centers. Add remaining ingredients to food processor and pulse until coarsely chopped. Pour mixture into pie dish and serve. You can heat to warm if you desire. Peel Apples and remove centers.

Strawberry Pie

- 2 cups almonds
- ½ cup dates
- 2 Tbsp ground flax seed
- 1 package fresh strawberries
- 2 ripe bananas
- 2 tsp fresh lemon juice
- 1 Tbsp Agave nectar

Crust: Soak 1/2 cup dates for 20 minutes and drain. Add almonds to food processor and pulse until large minced pieces. Add dates and ground flax seed. Pulse until mixture is blended and minced. Press into pie dish. Filling: Soak 1/2 cup dates for 20 minutes and drain. Add 1/2 package of strawberries to food processor. Add 1/2 cup soaked dates, agave, lemon juice and bananas and pulse until mixed together. Do not blend excessive. Leave small chunks. Pour into pie dish. Slice remaining strawberries and place on top of mixture. Serve chilled.

What is a good sugar substitute?

There are many good sugar substitutes. Let me start by saying do not use Aspartame or Saccharin. These are big time poisons to our body that is much worse than sugar itself. These sweeteners are found in NutriSweet products along with Equal and Canderel.

Stevia and Tagatose are my favorite sweeteners if you are going to use them. These both are all natural sweeteners with no chemical additives. Tagatose is the better of the two for cooking because it is created to use the same amount of volume as normal sugar whereas Stevia is much more potent and has a little bit of a licorice taste to it.

Lemon Squares

- ½ cup dates
- ½ cup pecans
- ½ cup walnuts
- ¾ cup almonds
- 3 Tbsp honey
- 2 Tbsp ground flax seed
- 1 cup cashews
- ½ cup shredded coconut flakes
- ¼ cup fresh lemon juice
- 2 Tbsp lemon zest
- 2 Tbsp Agave nectar

Crust: Soak 1/2 cup dates for 20 minutes and drain. Add almonds to food processor and process into a course flour. Add pecans, 1/2 cup soaked dates, walnuts, almonds and honey. Pulse until ingredients are minced and turn into a dough texture. Press into an 8 x 8 pan. Soak cashews for 20 minutes and drain. Soak dates for 20 minutes and drain. Add cashews, lemon juice, ground flax seed and soaked dates to blender and blend well. Pour over crust. Spread lemon Zest over filling. Spread coconut over filling. Best if chilled overnight.

What can I do for Holiday Meals?

I love Holiday meals because it lets me create all my favorites for one meal. If you really think about a Holiday, it has predominately plant based dishes nestled around a turkey or ham. Depending on who we are having over will depend if I actually cook a turkey or if I just create my favorite hot dish with 9 or 10 side dishes and 3 desserts. I can still waddle away from a holiday table without compromising. Another twist is to go ahead and allow yourself to have a feast. Just know that after this one meal (not after 15 turkey sandwiches with Mayo) that you are going to get back on the plant based diet. When we first started this, I would indulge with turkey or ham. After several holidays, I no longer care to indulge. There are all these other scrumptious dishes to choose from that the greasy bird just doesn't hold anything for me. If you are fighting cancer, then I recommend that you do not indulge. Your life is more important than one SAD meal.

Cheese Cake

- 2 cups almonds
- ½ cup dates
- ¼ cup shredded coconut flakes (optional)
- 3 cups cashews
- ¾ cup fresh lemon juice
- ¾ cup honey
- ½ cup coconut oil
- 1 ½ tsp vanilla
- ½ tsp sea salt
- ¼ cup water
- 1 cup frozen raspberries
- 2 Tbsp ground flax seed

Crust: Soak dates in water for 20 minutes and drain. Add soaked dates, almonds and ground flax seed to food processor and pulse until mixed and minced. Sprinkle coconut flakes in a spring form pan. Press mixture into pan bottom. Filling: Soak Cashews for 20 minutes and drain. Add soaked cashews, lemon juice, honey, coconut oil, vanilla, salt and water to a blender and blend very well for several minutes. Pour filling into pan and freeze for several hours. Topping: Soak dates for 20 minutes and drain. Add dates and frozen raspberries to food processor and pulse until chunky. Pour over cheesecake and serve.

Pumpkin Soufflé

- 4 grated sweet potatoes
- 1 cup dates
- 1 tsp vanilla
- 1 tsp cinnamon
- 1 tsp pumpkin spice
- 1 tsp sea salt
- 2 Tbsp coconut oil
- 3 cups water
- 2 tsp Psyllium
- 1 cup pecans
- ½ cup Agave nectar

Pit and soak dates for 20 minutes and drain. Peel sweet potatoes and using the grating blade in your food processor, grate 4 cups of sweet potato. Add all ingredients except pecans to a blender and blend very well for several minutes. Pour mixture into dish. Sprinkle pecans on top and chill.

Lori's German Chocolate Cake

Cake
- 2 Cups whole grain white flour
- 1 cup honey
- 3/4 cups carob
- 1 tsp baking soda
- 1 tsp baking powder
- 1/2 tsp sea salt
- 1 1/2 tsp vanilla
- 2 tsp vinegar
- 1/4 cup coconut milk
- 1 cup water
- 1/2 cup coconut flakes
- 1/2 Vegenaise
- 1 cup pecan pieces
- 1 cup walnut pieces
- 1/4 carob chips
- 2 Tbsp grape seed oil

Frosting
- 1 1/2 cups almonds
- 1 1/2 cups walnuts
- 1 1/2 cups dates
- 1 1/2 cups coconut flakes
- 3/4 cup agave nectar
- 2 Tbsp carob chips

Combine ingredients and bake at 340° for 35 minutes.

Carob Pudding

- ¼ cup coconut oil
- ½ cup Agave nectar
- ¾ cup carob powder
- ½ cup fresh squeezed orange juice
- 1 tsp orange zest
- ¼ tsp sea salt
- ½ cup toasted almonds
- ½ tsp vanilla
- 2 avocados

Add oil, carob, orange juice, agave, salt, vanilla and avocados to blender and blend well. Toast almonds in oven until golden brown. Spoon pudding into 4 dishes. Top with orange zest and almonds. Chill and serve.

Carob Almond Truffles

- ½ cup honey
- 1 cup uncooked oatmeal
- 2 tsp ground flax seed
- 1 cup almond butter
- 1 Tbsp coconut oil
- 1 tsp vanilla
- ½ cup carob powder
- ½ tsp sea salt
- ½ cashew pieces

Mix dry ingredients well. Melt coconut butter. Add remaining ingredients except cashews. Roll mixture into ½" balls. Using the S blade in your food processor, mince cashews. Roll carob balls in cashew pieces. Chill and serve.

Keylime Pudding

- 3 avocados
- 1 ripe banana
- 1 mango
- ¾ cup keylime juice (about 15 keylimes)
- 1 tsp lime zest
- ½ cup Agave nectar
- ¼ cup coconut oil
- 1 ½ tsp vanilla
- ½ tsp sea salt

Place all ingredients except zest into blender and blend until smooth. Pour pudding into 6 dishes. Sprinkle zest on top. Chill and serve.

MISCELLANEOUS

What are good snacks?

A favorite snack for me is Pineapple. It is wonderfully sweet and has so many good nutrients and trace minerals. It has Bromelain, an enzyme that is great for anti-inflammatory and anti-mucus. Buy fresh pineapple and keep it in your refrigerator. If it starts to get old, just plop it in your smoothies.

Bananas are another favorite of mine. Bananas are packed with Potassium. Potassium is great for cardiovascular health and bone health. It is also a complex carbohydrate that will keep giving you energy for a long time. Try to not snack on nuts. Nuts are very high in calories and fat. It is easy to eat too many nuts if you use them as a snack.

Refried Beans

- 2 cups dried pinto beans
- 2 Tbsp garlic powder
- 2 Tbsp sea salt
- 2 Tbsp coconut oil
- 1 Tbsp onion powder
- ½ tsp cayenne powder
- 6 cups water

Cook pinto beans until very tender. Add remaining ingredients. Take 3/4 of beans and blend in blender until smooth. Mix with remaining beans.

Cheese Sauce

- 1 cup vegenaise
- 1/3 cup nutritional yeast

Mix together. Use for macaroni or add 1/4 cup water and use as cheese sauce.

Thousand Island Dressing

- 1 cup vegenaise
- 1 fresh lemon – juiced
- 2 Tbsp raw Agave nectar or honey
- 1 stalk of celery
- ½ cup sun dried tomatoes
- ½ tsp onion powder
- 1/3 cup water

Place sun dried tomatoes in 1/3 cup of water for 20 minutes. Add water and sundried tomatoes and all ingredients to blender and blend well.

Ranch Dressing

- 1 cup vegenaise
- 1 tsp garlic powder
- 1 Tbsp onion powder
- 1 tsp Italian seasoning
- 1 fresh lemon – juiced
- ½ tsp sea salt
- ¼ tsp celery salt
- ¼ cup water

Mix all ingredients together and let sit for 15 minutes to blend flavors.

Guacamole

- 3 ripe avocados
- 1 fresh lime – juiced
- 1 clove garlic – minced
- ¼ head lettuce – finely minced
- ¼ sweet onion – finely minced
- ¼ tsp sea salt
- 1 Jalapeño – finely minced

Put lettuce, onion, garlic, jalapeño and lime juice in blender and pulse until minced. Using a fork smash the peeled avocados to a mush. Add remaining ingredients. To preserve, cover tightly with saran wrap.

Sweet Onion Salad Dressing

- ½ sweet onion
- 1/3 cup honey
- ½ cup apple cider vinegar
- 1 Tbsp Dijon mustard
- 1/3 cup grape seed oil or olive oil
- 1 tsp poppy seeds

Place all ingredients in blender and blend well.

Italian Nut Cheese Spread

- 1 cup pine nuts
- 2 cloves garlic
- ½ tsp onion powder
- ¼ cup fresh basil or 2 Tbsp dried
- ½ cup distilled water
- ½ tsp sea salt

Soak almonds for 1 hour. Place almonds in a blender and blend with water until creamy. Strain almond cream through a cheese cloth. Place almond meat in bowl and add additional ingredients.

High Protein Salad Dressing

- ½ cup sunflower seeds
- 1 stalk of celery
- 3 cloves garlic
- ¼ cup fresh cilantro
- 2 Tbsp apple cider vinegar
- 2 Tbsp honey
- 1 tsp Braggs Aminos
- ½ cup water

Place all ingredients in blender and blend well.

Garlic Dressing

- 10 cloves garlic
- ¼ cup fresh lemon juice
- ¾ cup apple cider vinegar
- 1 tsp sea salt
- 1 Tbsp dried parsley
- 1 cup grape seed oil or olive oil
- 2 cups water
- 1 cup pine nuts
- 1 Tbsp Agave nectar

Add all ingredients together and blend well.

Mango Salsa

- 1 tomato
- 1 mango
- 1/4 sweet onion
- 1/2 green bell pepper
- Minced fresh jalapeno to taste
- 1 tsp agave nectar

Dice all ingredients and mix together.

Dehydrated Kale Chips

- 3 bunches of kale
- ½ cup apple cider vinegar
- 2 Tbsp Braggs Aminos
- 1/3 cup nutritional yeast flakes
- 1 Tbsp garlic powder
- 1 Tbsp onion powder

Remove kale leaves from stems. Holding the kale tightly together cut kale into 1/2" size pieces. In a large bowl combine tahini, vinegar, Braggs, yeast flakes ,garlic and onion powder. Massage kale into liquid. Place kale on dehydrator sheets and sprinkle with additional nutritional yeast. Place in dehydrator at 105 degrees for 8 hours or until crispy.

Healthy Oatmeal

- 3 cups oatmeal
- ½ cup walnuts
- ½ cup raisins or craisins
- ½ tsp sea salt
- 4 ½ cups water

Heat water on stove (not microwave), mince walnuts. Add walnuts, raisins and salt to oatmeal. Pour hot water into oatmeal and let stand 1 minute. You can also add cinnamon or diced apple and a little bit of agave or honey to sweeten your oatmeal.

Blue Cheese Flavor Dressing

- 2 Tbsp Braggs Aminos
- 2 Tbsp apple cider vinegar
- 3 Tbsp nutritional yeast flakes
- 1 tsp onion powder
- 1 tsp garlic powder
- ½ tsp sea salt
- ½ cup grape seed oil or olive oil
- 3 Tbsp vegenaise

Place all ingredients in blender and blend well.